Textbook of
Pharmaceutical Calculation
and
Extemporaneous
Preparations

Based on New PCI Syllabus

for **BPharm, Biotechnology and Basic Sciences**

Textbook of
Pharmaceutical Calculation
and
Extemporaneous Preparations

Based on New PCI Syllabus

for **BPharm, Biotechnology and Basic Sciences**

HK Sharma
MPharm (Pharmaceutics), PhD
Associate Professor
Department of Pharmaceutical Sciences
Dibrugarh University, Dibrugarh, Assam
Email:hemantasharma123@yahoo.co.in

Nayanmoni Boruah
MPharm (Pharmaceutics)
Department of Pharmaceutical Sciences
Dibrugarh University, Dibrugarh, Assam
Email:boruahnayanmoni1@gmail.com

CBSPD

CBS Publishers & Distributors Pvt Ltd

New Delhi • Bengaluru • Chennai • Kochi • Kolkata • Lucknow • Mumbai
Hyderabad • Jharkhand • Nagpur • Patna • Pune • Uttarakhand

Textbook of
Pharmaceutical Calculation
and
**Extemporaneous
Preparations**

ISBN: 978-93-88178-91-4

Copyright © Authors and Publisher

First Edition: 2019

Reprint: 2022, 2024

Published by Satish Kumar Jain and Produced by Varun Jain for

CBS Publishers & Distributors Pvt Ltd

4819/XI Prahlad Street, 24 Ansari Road, Daryaganj, New Delhi 110 002, India
Ph: 011-23289259, 23266861   Website: www.cbspd.com
                                    e-mail: delhi@cbspd.com
Corporate Office: 204 FIE, Industrial Area, Patparganj, Delhi 110 092
Ph: 011-4934 4934   Fax: 011-4934 4935   e-mail: publishing@cbspd.com; publicity@cbspd.com

Branches

- **Bengaluru:** Seema House 2975, 17th Cross, K.R. Road, Banasankari 2nd Stage, Bengaluru 560 070, Karnataka, India
  Ph: +91-80-26771678/79   Fax: +91-80-26771680   e-mail: bangalore@cbspd.com
- **Chennai:** 7, Subbaraya Street, Shenoy Nagar, Chennai 600 030, Tamil Nadu, India
  Ph: +91-44-26680620, 26681266   Fax: +91-44-42032115   e-mail: chennai@cbspd.com
- **Kochi:** 42/1325, 1326, Power House Road, Opp KSEB, Power House, Ernakulam 682 018, Kerala, India
  Ph: +91-484-4059061-65   Fax: +91-484-4059065   e-mail: kochi@cbspd.com
- **Kolkata:** 147, Hind Ceramics Compound, 1st Floor, Nilgunj Road, Belghoria, Kolkata-700056 West Bengal, India
  Ph: 033-25633055, 033-25633056   e-mail: kolkata@cbspd.com
- **Lucknow:** Basement, Khushnuma Complex, 7-Meerabai Marg (Behind Jawahar Bhawan) Lucknow 226001, India
  Ph: 0522-4000032   e-mail: tiwari.lucknow@cbspd.com
- **Mumbai:** PWD Shed. Gala no. 25/26, Ramchandra Bhatt Marg, Next to JJ Hospital Gate no. 2, Opp. Union Bank of India Noorbaug Mumbai-400009, Maharashtra, India
  Ph: 022-66661880/89   e-mail: mumbai@cbspd.com

Representatives

- **Hyderabad** 0-9885175004
- **Jharkhand** 0-9811541605
- **Nagpur** 0-8692091830
- **Patna** 0-9334159340
- **Pune** 0-9664372571
- **Uttarakhand** 0-9716462459

Printed at Rashtriya Printers, Dilshad Garden, Delhi, India

Foreword

About ten years ago, when I was working as a scientist at the Centre for Cellular and Molecular Biology (CSIR), Hyderabad, one MSc student came to work for two months in my project as a part of the summer training program of CCMB. On the very first day, I gave him the composition of a bacteriological medium. The concentration of the individual components were mentioned in terms of weight by volume (w/v) in the formula. I asked him to calculate the amount needed of each component to make a 500 ml solution. True to my anticipation, he could not do it. I admonished him and subsequently explained to him the method to calculate. The student successfully completed his project work and later on got authorship of a paper published by me. He passed MSc and also obtained PhD from the Delhi University. A couple of years ago, when he came to see me at CCMB as a lecturer of a college in Delhi, he recollected the calculation that he learnt from me on the first day of his training program and mentioned that he had preserved the record book with the calculation on its first page.

His inability to make such a simple calculation was deplorable but not an isolated case. I have come across many research scholars and even a few scientists, belonging to the same category. They do not understand the basics, needed to prepare a solution by weighing and dissolving individual components, to get the correct amount required to inject to an experimental animal or to prepare a buffer with the desired pH. Being fully aware that the ineptitude for such a simple job is not expected from a person of their experience and designation, they hesitate to approach anybody for help in learning the basic calculations, essential for laboratory work.

Against this backdrop, the monograph prepared by Dr HK Sharma and his student Mr Nayanmoni Boruah, appears to be of immense help to the pharmacy professionals, researchers and students alike, to get acquainted with the basic knowledge essential for laboratory works. One, having the book in his possession, need not seek help from anybody for preparing the reagents for an experiment. Dr Sharma was a very hard working and sincere student all through his academic career. He has prepared this book with meticulous care. He has rightly appreciated the problems; a beginner is likely to be confronted with, in making an experimental set-up and has explained the procedures with relevant examples. Inter-conversion of one unit of the strength of a solution into another unit is a task, most often required for dilution of stock solutions. Dr Sharma has demonstrated and explained all types of calculations, needed for this purpose. Preparation of emulsions and multi-component dry powders is also a routine job in pharmaceutical practice. Dr Sharma has explained the protocols in a very lucid manner. He has also demonstrated the basic calculations, required for routine works in microbiology. The list of Latin expressions, most often seen in prescriptions, with meaning makes the book very useful. I hope this book will be widely circulated in the laboratories, academic institutions as well as pharmaceutical and chemical companies, located all over the country.

MK Chattopadhyay MPharm, PhD

Senior Principal Scientist (Retired)
Centre for Cellular and Molecular Biology (CSIR)
Hyderabad, India

Preface

This book is a high-priority textbook designed to meet the needs of the students of bachelor of pharmacy course. This book aims to build the foundation stone for pharmacy students. As pharmaceutical calculations are involved in pharmaceutics, pharmaceutical analysis, pharmacognosy and pharmacology, this book will guide students to acquire the basic pharmaceutical calculation concepts. Examples are included in each chapter, which will help students understand the problems. This book covers many chapters of pharmaceutics I theory paper as well as the whole syllabus of pharmaceutics 1 practical paper as per the new syllabus for B Pharm course. It also partly covers the syllabus for Pharmaceutics V practical paper. All chapters are explained with examples so that students can easily understand every topic. For self-assessment purpose, many questions are included at the end of each chapter. comprehensive list of physiological units will be useful for students of pharmacy as well as allied branches including basic sciences and biotechnology. Physical units and their conversion is a unique addition to the book. The description of pharmaceutical preparations (extemporaneous preparations) would be helpful in selecting preparations from different categories. Although, extemporaneous preparations are seldom used in pharmacy practice, however, the description would help students to understand the concept of formulation.

Pharmaceutical calculation is a fundamental part of pharmaceutical sciences. The basic knowledge of pharmaceutical calculation is necessary to understand and deal with pharmaceutical problems starting from chemical analysis to pharmaceutical formulation. There is a need for a systematic approach to understand every topic related to the pharmaceutical calculation at the beginning of the journey. There are a few books which cover various topics of pharmaceutical calculation in a single book. Due to tremendous development in pharmaceutical sciences and continuous revision of syllabus for pharmacy students, there is a need for a pharmaceutical calculation book, which can be used as a textbook as well as a reference book. Keeping this need of the students in mind, this book has been compiled in such a manner that it will provide all the necessary chapters related to pharmaceutical calculation as well as extemporaneous preparations.

Considering the needs of students, we have made every possible effort to ensure accuracy of data and illustrations provided in this book and also prioritized incorporation of important topics. However, incorporation of more calculation based topics would have fulfilled the needs of students and researchers of pharmacy and allied branches. We will ensure, the future editions will meet these requirements.

HK Sharma
Nayanmoni Boruah

Acknowledgement

Designing and planning of a textbook, on any subject is a difficult task due to changing syllabic content. There must be appropriate feelings and understanding of the needs of students. Students discuss and convey their needs to teachers and therefore, I am thankful to all the students, who discussed and expressed their needs to me.

I also thankful to the team of CBS Publishers & Distributors Pvt Ltd, New Delhi, for their interest, support and cooperation in publishing this book for the benefit of students.

HK Sharma

Contents

1 Pharmaceutical Measurement System

Measurement is the basic knowledge of all technical operations in pharmaceutical sector. Pharmacy students must be aware of different pharmaceutical measurement systems. They must also know the measurement of weights and volumes in different measurement systems.

Three measurement systems are well known in pharmaceutical sector and commonly used worldwide. These systems are:

  i. Metric system
 ii. Apothecaries system
iii. Avoirdupois system

METRIC SYSTEM

The idea of adopting a standard scientific measurement system was suggested by a number of scientists during seventeenth-century such as French astronomer Jean Picard, Scottish inventor James Watt. The metric system was formulated during late eighteen century in French. United States legalized use of metric system in 1866. United States of Pharmacopoeia, 1890, adopted the metric system of weights and measures. British Pharmacopoeia, 1914, adopted the metric system of weights and measures. Due to simplicity and adaptability, metric system is the most widely used popular measurement system. The present standards of metric system are defined in publications of the National Institute of Standards and Technology (NIST).

FRACTION AND MULTIPLE PREFIXES

Pharmaceutical calculation frequently includes very small quantity of length, weight, time, and volume or radioactivity measurement. Expression of these small quantities involves use of numbers with many zeros. This expression may lead to error in calculation. To avoid this, NIST recognizes prefixes to express fractions or multiples of SI units.

Table 1.1 Prefix and symbol

Multiple	Prefix	Symbol	Submultiple	Prefix	Symbol
10^{24}	yotta	Y	10^{-1}	deci	d
10^{21}	zetta	Z	10^{-2}	centi	c
10^{18}	Exa	E	10^{-3}	milli	m
10^{15}	peta	P	10^{-6}	micro	µ
10^{12}	tera	T	10^{-9}	nano	n
10^{9}	giga	G	10^{-12}	pico	P
10^{6}	mega	M	10^{-15}	femto	f
10^{3}	kilo	k	10^{-18}	atto	a
10^{2}	hecto	h	10^{-21}	zepto	z
10	deca	da	10^{-24}	yocto	y

Table 1.2 Prefix and factor

Power	Factor	prefix
10^{18}	1000000000000000000	exa
10^{15}	1000000000000000	peta
10^{12}	1000000000000	tera
10^{9}	1000000000	giga
10^{6}	1000000	mega
10^{3}	1000	kilo
10^{2}	100	hecto
10	10	deca
10^{0}	1	–
10^{-1}	0.1	deci
10^{-2}	0.01	centi
10^{-3}	0.001	milli
10^{-6}	0.000001	micro
10^{-9}	0.000000001	nano
10^{-12}	0.000000000001	pico
10^{-15}	0.000000000000001	femto
10^{-18}	0.000000000000000001	atto

Table 1.3 Metric weight measurement

Weight in different units	Symbol	Weight in gram
1 nanogram	ng	10^{-9} g
1 microgram	μg	10^{-6} g
1 milligram	mg	10^{-3} g
1 centigram	cg	10^{-2} g
1 decigram	dg	10^{-1} g
1 gram	g	1 g
1 dekagram	dag	10 g
1 hectogram	hg	10^{2} g
1 kilogram	kg	10^{3} g

Table 1.4 Metric volume measurement

Volume in different units	Symbol	Volume in litre
1 kilolitre	kL	10^{3} L
1 hectolitre	hL	10^{2} L
1 dekalitre	daL	10 L
1 litre	L	1 L
1 decilitre	dL	10^{-1} L
1 centilitre	cL	10^{-2} L
1 millilitre	mL	10^{-3} L
1 microlitre	μL	10^{-6} L

Table 1.5 Metric linear measurement

Length in different units	Symbol	Length in metre
1 kilometre	km	10^{3} m
1 hectometre	hm	10^{2} m
1 dekametre	dam	10 m
1 metre	m	1 m
1 decimetre	dm	10^{-1} m
1 centimetre	cm	10^{-2} m
1 millimetre	mm	10^{-3} m
1 micrometre	μm	10^{-6} m
1 nanometre	nm	10^{-9} m

Metric system consists of three variants. These variants are:

1. Centimetre-gram-second system (CGS)
2. Metre-kilogram-second system (MKS)
3. Metre-tonne-second system (MTS)

International System of Units, SI was established by General Conference on Weights and Measures (CGPM). SI units are defined by CGPM. It is an extension of MKS system. The base quantities used in SI are mass, time, length, electric current, thermodynamic temperature, amount of substance and luminous intensity.

Table 1.6 Base quantities and base units used in SI

Base quantity	Symbol for quantity	Symbol for dimension	Unit name	Symbol for unit
Length	l, x, r	L	metre	m
Mass	M	M	kilogram	kg
Time, duration	T	T	second	s
Electric current	I, i	I	ampere	A
Thermodynamic temperature	T	Θ	kelvin	K
Amount of substance	N	N	mole	mol
Luminous intensity	I_v	J	candela	cd

Table 1.7 Few non-SI units accepted for use with SI units

Quantity	Name of unit	Symbol for unit	Values in SI unit
Mass	tonne	T	$10^3\,kg$
Volume	litre	L, l	$10^{-3}\,m^3$
Area	hectare	ha	$10^4\,m^2$
Plane angle	degree	°	$1° = (\pi/180)$ rad
	minute	′	$1' = (\pi/10800)$ rad
	second	″	$1'' = (\pi/648000)$ rad
Time	minute	min	60 s
	hour	h	3600 s
	day		86400

DEFINITION OF BASE UNITS (AS GIVEN BY BIPM, 2008)

1. *Unit of length (metre):* The metre is the length of the path travelled by light in vacuum during a time interval of 1/299792458 of a second.

2. *Unit of mass (kilogram):* The kilogram is the unit of mass; it is equal to the mass of the international prototype of the kilogram.

3. *Unit of time (second):* The second is the duration of 9192631770 periods of the radiation corresponding to the transition between the two hyperfine levels of the ground state of the caesium 133 atom. This definition refers to a caesium atom at rest at a temperature of $0\,°K$.

4. *Unit of electric current (ampere):* The ampere is that constant current which, if maintained in two straight parallel conductors of infinite length, of negligible circular cross-section, and placed 1 metre apart in vacuum, would produce between these conductors a force equal to 2×10^{-7} newton per metre of length.

5. *Unit of thermodynamic temperature (kelvin):* The kelvin, unit of thermodynamic temperature, is the fraction $1/273.16$ of the thermodynamic temperature of the triple point of water. This definition refers to water having the isotopic composition defined exactly by the following amount of substance ratios: 0.00015576 mole of ^2H per mole of ^1H, 0.0003799 mole of ^{17}O per mole of ^{16}O, and 0.0020052 mole of ^{18}O per mole of ^{16}O.

6. *Unit of amount of substance (mole):* The mole is the amount of substance of a system which contains as many elementary entities as there are atoms in 0.012 kilogram of carbon 12; its symbol is "mol". When the mole is used, the elementary entities should be specified which may be atoms, molecules, ions, electrons, other particles, or specified groups of such particles.

7. *Unit of luminous intensity (candela):* Candela is the unit of luminous intensity, in a given direction, of a source that emits monochromatic radiation of frequency 540×1012 hz and that has a radiant intensity in that direction of $1/683$ watt per steradian.

RULES AND STYLE CONVENTIONS FOR USING SI UNITS

1. *Typeface:* Unit symbols should be printed in roman (upright) type.

2. *Capitalization:* Unit symbols are written in lower case letters. Exceptions are:

   a. The unit symbol or first letter of the unit symbol is an upper-case letter when its name is derived from the name of the scientist

   b. In case of symbol for litre, L is also used.

3. *Plurals:* Unit symbols should be used as per the given rule. It must be unaltered in plural.

   > *Example:* Length = 50 cm (correct)
   >
   > Length = 50 cms (incorrect)

4. *Punctuation:* Unit symbols must not followed by period unless at the end of the complete sentence.

   > *Example:* This scale is 50 cm long. (correct)
   >
   > This scale is 50 cm. long. (incorrect)

5. *Multiplication of symbols:* Symbols for units which are formed by multiplication of other units should be expressed by indicating the multiplication with a half high dot or space.

   Example:

   > $m \cdot s^{-1}$ or $m\ s^{-1}$ (It means metre per second)
   >
   > ms^{-1} (It is the symbol for reciprocal of millisecond)

6. *Division of symbols:* Symbols for units which are formed by division of other units can be expressed in the following ways:

   - m/s, $\dfrac{m}{s}$ or $m \cdot s^{-1}$ (correct)
   - m/s^2 or $m \cdot s^{-2}$ (correct)
     $m/s/s$ (incorrect)
   - $m \cdot kg/(s^3 \cdot A)$ or $m\ kg \cdot s^{-3} \cdot A^{-1}$ (correct)
     $m \cdot kg/s^3/A$ (incorrect)

7. *Unit name and unit symbol:* Unit name and unit symbol should not be used together.

   Example: C/kg or coulomb per kilogram (correct)
   Coulomb/kg, coulomb per kg, C/kilogram, coulomb kg^{-1}, C per kg, coulomb/kilogram (incorrect)

8. *Abbreviation of units:* Abbreviation should not be used for unit symbols or unit name. Some of them are:

Unit name	Unit symbol	Abbreviations (should not be used)
Second	s	sec
Square millimetre	mm^2	mm
Hours	h	hrs
Minutes	min	mins
Litre	L	lit
Atomic mass unit	u	amu

RULES AND STYLE CONVENTIONS FOR USING SI PREFIXES

1. *Typeface:* Prefix should be attached to unit symbol without a space. Prefix name and nit symbol should be printed in roman (upright) type.

   Example: pm (picometre), THz (tetrahertz)

2. *Capitalization:* The prefix symbol should be written in upper case letter for Y (yotta), Z (zetta), E (exa), P (peta), T (tera), G (giga), and M (mega) and for others in lower case letter as given in Table 1.1.

3. *Inseparability of prefix and unit:* Prefix name and unit name is separable in the case where they are attached together. Such as nm (nanometre), but it should not be written as mµm (millimicrometre).

4. *Use of multiple prefixes:* When prefix symbols are present in both numerator and denominator, it is better express only one of the symbols with prefix to avoid confusion.

   Example: 10 MV · ms is acceptable but 10 kV · s is more preferable.

5. Prefix symbol should not be used alone.

   Example: $6 \times 10^{12}/m^3$ (correct)

   $6 \, T/m^3$ (incorrect)

6. Prefix symbols should not be used with angle related symbols and time related symbols to avoid confusion.

RULES FOR EXPRESSING VALUES FOR QUANTITIES

1. The product of a number and unit is called value of a quantity and the number multiplying the unit is known as numerical value for the quantity.
2. A space is left between numerical value and unit symbol in the expression of value of a quantity.
   Example: $T = 50\,°C$ (correct) $T = 50\,°C$ or $50\,°C$ (incorrect)
3. The value of a quantity can be expressed using only one unit.
   Length = 5.196 m (correct)
   Length = 5 m 19 cm 6 mm (incorrect)
4. Information must not be attached to unit.
   Example: $V_{max} = 500\ V$ (correct)
   $V = 500\ V_{max}$ (should not be used)
5. Information should not be mixed with units.
   Example:
   a. Al content 10 ng/L (correct)
      10 ng Al/L or 10 ng of aluminum/L (incorrect)
   b. Electron emission rate is $2 \times 10^{15}/s$ (correct)
      Emission rate is $2 \times 10^{15}\ e/s$ (incorrect)
   c. The number density of He atoms is $5 \times 10^{22}/cm^3$ (correct)
   The number density is 5×10^{22} He atoms/ cm^3 (correct)
6. Symbol for number and units should be used.
7. Symbols, numbers and units should be used instead spelled out names for numbers and units.
   Length of the tube is 10 cm (correct)
   Length of the tube is ten centimetre (should not be used)
8. Clarity in writing:
   25 cm × 25 cm × 25 cm (correct)
   25 × 25 × 25 cm (incorrect)
   200 nm to 400 nm or (200 to 400) nm (correct)
   200 to 400 nm or 200–400 nm (incorrect)
   25.1 cm ± 0.5 cm or (25.1 ± 0.5) cm (correct)
   25.1 ± 0.5 cm or 25.1 cm ± 0.5 (incorrect)

9. Stand-alone unit symbol should not be used.

   Without numerical values or quantity symbols, symbols for units should not be used.

   There are 10^3 ml in 1 L (correct)

   There are many ml in a L (unacceptable)

10. Selection of SI prefixes:

    Selection of SI prefixes depends on several factors. These factors include

    a. Numerical value should be easily understood

    b. Indication of digits of a numerical value which are significant

    c. Practice in the particular field of science and technology

    Prefix symbols should be selected in such a way that numerical values lies between 0.1 and 1000, and prefix symbols should represent the number 10 raised to a power of multiple of 3.

    Example: 4.9×10^{-8} g may be written as 49×10^{-9} g = 49 ng

11. Use of percentage symbol:

    A space should be left between the symbol % and numerical value.

    Example:

    $X_A = 0.0031 = 3.1$ % (correct)

    $X_A = 0.0031 = 3.1$% or 0.25 percent (incorrect)

    X_A – Quantity symbol (amount of substance fraction of A)

12 ppm, ppb and ppt symbols are not acceptable in SI system.

13. Roman numerals should not be used to express numerical values. Such one must not use M as substitutes for 10^3.

14. "Divided by" or "per" rather than the words "per unit" should be used in case of derived units which are formed by division of other units.

    Example: Pressure is force divided by area or pressure is force per area (correct)

    Pressure is force per unit area (incorrect)

15. While reporting the value of a quantity, one must distinguish between a substance and an attribute which is ascribed to the substance. Such as a surface and its area, an object and its mass.

Note: Rules related to expression of SI units recommended by NIST are generally followed; however, deviations are also observed. For example: In official pharmacopoeia

i. Dose of a drug is expressed as 2–4 mg or 2 to 4 mg.

ii. While using % symbol, in official pharmacopoeias, % w/w or % v/v is written.

These are two examples of deviation from the suggestions of NIST. The deviations are also found to be discipline specific, hence, similar examples may be observed in other disciplines also.

Example: An object of mass 15 kg, loaded into the granulator.

Table 1.8	Greek alphabet in Roman	
Greek alphabet character	*Roman type*	
	Upper case letter	*Lower case letter*
Alpha	A	α
Beta	B	β
Gamma	Γ	γ
Delta	Δ	δ
Epsilon	E	ε
Zeta	Z	ζ
Eta	H	η
Theta	Θ	θ
Iota	I	ι
Kappa	K	κ
Lambda	Λ	λ
Mu	M	μ
Nu	N	ν
Xi	Ξ	ξ
Omicron	O	ο
Pi	Π	π
Rho	P	ρ
Sigma	Σ	σ
Tau	T	τ
Upsilon	Y	υ
Phi	Φ	φ
Chi	X	χ
Psi	Ψ	ψ
Omega	Ω	ω

APOTHECARIES' SYSTEM OF MEASUREMENT

Apothecary system is used for compounding and dispensing of drugs. This system originates from troy weight system. London College of Physicians, adopted troy weight in 1618 on recommendation of Sir Theodore Turquet de la Mayerne, compiler of their first pharmacopoiea. All apothecaries under British customs have started buying and selling of medicines under *avoirdupois system* and compounding them by *apothecary system*. In spite of increasing popularity of metric system, other systems are still prevelant.

Table 1.9 Apothecaries' weight measurement

Pound (lb)	Ounce (℥)	Drachm (ℨ)	Scurple (℈)	Grain (gr.)
1	12	96	288	5760
	1	8	24	480
		1	3	60
			1	20

Table 1.10 Apothecaries' fluid measurement

Gallon (gal.)	Quart (qt.)	Pint (pt.)	Fluid ounce (℥)	Fluidrachm (f ℨ)	Minim (♏)
1	4	8	128	1024	61440
	1	2	32	256	3840
		1	16	128	7680
			1	8	480
				1	60

AVOIRDUPOIS

Avoirdupois is a measurement which has been used for buying and selling medicines.

Table 1.11 Avoirdupois weight measurement system

Pound (lb)	Ounce (oz.)	Grain (gr.)
1	16	7000
	1	437.5

Table 1.12	Imperial measurement of liquid (British)			
Gallon	Pint	Fluid ounce	Fluidrachm	Minim
1	8	160	1280	76800
	1	20	160	9600
		1	8	480
			1	60

PRACTICAL EQUIVALENTS

Equivalents of linear measure
1 metre = 39.4 inches
1 inch = 2.54 cm

Equivalents of liquid measure
(Apothecary)
1 ml = 16.23 minims
1 minim = 0.0616 ml
1 fluidrachm = 3.96 ml
1 fluid ounce = 29.57 ml
1 pint = 473 ml
1 gallon = 3785 ml
1 gallon = 128 fluid ounces
1 fluid ounce (water)
= 455 grain

Equivalents of weight measure
1 grain (avoirdupois)
= 0.065 g
1 g = 15.432 grain
1 lb (avoirdupois) = 454 g
1 lb (apothecary) = 373.2 g
1 ounce (apothecary)
= 31.1 g

Table 1.13	Conversion of household measurement to approximate metric measures	
Household measurement	Apothecary notation	Metric volume
1 teaspoonful	f𝟹i	4 ml
1 dessertspoonful	f𝟹ii	8 ml
1 tablespoonful	f℥ss	15 ml
1 wineglassful	f℥ ii	60 ml
1 teacupful	f℥iv	120 ml
1 tumblerful	f℥viii	240 ml

SMALLEST WEIGHABLE QUANTITY

Sensitivity of balances plays an important role in weighing. If a balance has sensitivity requirement of 5 mg, then maximum potential error is ±4 mg.

Percentage of error can be defined as

$$\text{Percentage of error} = \frac{\text{Error} \times 100\%}{\text{Quantity desired}}$$

Therefore, more amount of weighed quantity means low percentage of error.

To find out the minimum weighable quantity, we must know maximum permissible percentage of error and sensitivity requirement of the balance. United States of Pharmacopoeia allows 5 percent error.

$$\text{Minimum weighable} = \frac{\substack{\text{Maximum potential error} \\ \text{or sensitvity requirement} \times 100}}{\text{Permissible percentage of error}}$$

2 Latin Terms and Their Use in Prescription

LATIN TERMS

Latin terms and their use in prescription

Latin words are used in prescription basically, for four reasons:

1. These words are not susceptible to change in the meaning of the word as compared to other languages used in daily use as the Latin language is virtually dead.
2. The prescription can be easily understood by physician and pharmacist belong to different places or nations.
3. The Latin names of medicinal plants and other objects are definite and there is no risk of misinterpretation.
4. Latin terms and abbreviations provide technical secrecy to a great extent.

Classification of Latin terms according to their use in prescription

1. Latin terms and abbreviations related to body parts.
2. Latin terms and abbreviations related to dosage forms.
3. Latin terms and abbreviations related to time of administration.
4. Numerical terms.
5. Miscellaneous Latin terms and abbreviations.

Latin terms and abbreviations related to body parts

Latin term	Abbreviation	Meaning
Brachio	Brach.	To the arm
Capiti	–	To the head
Corpori	Corp.	To the body
Cruri	–	To the leg
Dolente parti	Dolent. Part.	To the affected part
In aurem sinistram	In aur. sinist	To the left ear
In oculum dextrum	In ocul. dext	Into the right eye
In singulos aureus	In sng. Aur.	Into each ear
Jugulo	Jug.	To the throat
Mamma	–	To the breast
Naso	–	To the nose
Oculo	Ocul.	To the eye, for the eye
Procapillis	Pro. capill	For the hair
Pro singulas oculis	Pro. Sing. Ocul.	For each eye

Latin terms and abbreviations related to dosage forms

Latin term	Abbreviation	Meaning
Auristillae	auristill	The ear drops
Capsula	Caps.	A capsule
Cataplasma	Cataplasm.	A poultice
Cereolus	Cereol.	An urethral bougie
Charta	Chart.	A powder
Collunarium	Collun.	A nose wash
collutorium	Collut.	A mouth wash
collyrium	Collyr.	An eye lotion
Cremor	Crem.	A cream
Emplastrum	Emp.	A plaster
Emulsio	Emul.	An emulsion
Enema	–	An enema
Gargarisma	Garg.	A gargle
Guttae	Gtt.	Drops
Inhalatio	Inhal.	An inhalation
Injectio	Inj.	An injection
Linctus	Linct.	A linctus
Linimentum	Lin.	A liniment
Lotio	Lot.	A lotion

Contd...

Latin term	Abbreviation	Meaning
Mistura	m., mist	A mixture
Nebula	Neb.	A spray solution
Pasta	Past.	A paste
Pessus	Pess.	A pessary
Pgmentum	Pigm.	A paint
Pilula	Pil.	A pill
Pulvis	Pulv.	A powder
Suppositorium	Suppos.	A suppository
Tabella	Tab.	A tablet
trochiscus	Troch.	A lozenge
Unguentum	Ung.	An ointment

Latin terms and abbreviations related to time of administration

Latin term	Abbreviation	Meaning
Semel in die/semel die	Sem. in die/sem.die	Once a day
Indies/quotide	Indies/quot	daily
Bis in die/bis die	b. i. d./b. d.	Twice a day
Ter in die/Ter die	t. i. d./t. d.	Three times a day
Quarter in die/quarter die	q. d.	Four times a day
Primo mane	Prim. M.	Early in the morning
Omni mane	o. m.	Every morning
Jentaculum	Jentac	Breakfast
Meridie	–	Noon
Vespere	Vesp.	In the evening
Nocte	n.	At night
Omni nocte	o. n.	Every night
Horasomni	h. s.	At bed time
Hodie	–	To day
Cras	–	Tomorrow
Omni hora	o. h.	Every hour
Omni alternate hora	o. alt. h.	Every alternate hour
Ante meridiem	a. m.	Before noon
Post meritiem	p. m.	After noon
Ante cibum	a. c.	Before food
Post cibum	p. c.	After food
Doloreurgente	Dol. Urg.	When the pain is severe
Si opus sit	s. o. s.	When needed or when required
Statim	Stat.	Immediately

Miscellaneous Latin terms and abbreviations

Latin term	Abbreviation	Meaning
Ad	–	To, up to
Adde	Add	Add, let it be added
Admove	Admov.	apply
Aqua bulliens	Aq. Bull.	Boiling water
Aqua	Aq.	water
Capiat	Cap.	Let the patient take

3

Percentage Preparations

SOLVING PROBLEMS RELATED TO PERCENTAGE PREPARATIONS

Problems related to percentage weight in volume

To find out the percentage weight in volume of solute in the preparation when weight of solute and volume of preparation is provided.

Q. *Find out the percentage of a solution of dextrose, if 60 ml contain 3 g of dextrose?*

Solution:

60 ml solution contain 3 g of dextrose

Therefore, 100 ml of solution will contain $= \dfrac{3 \times 100}{60}$

$= 5$ g of dextrose

Percentage of dextrose in the given solution $= 5\%$ w/v

Alternative method

Density of water is almost 1 g/ml.

So, we can consider 60 ml of water is equal to 60 g of water.

60 g is equivalent to the 100% w/w of the solution; let us consider 3 g is equivalent to $x \%$ w/w.

$$\frac{x}{100} = \frac{3}{60}$$

$$x(\% \text{ w/w}) = \frac{3 \times 100}{60} = 5\% \text{ w/w}$$

To find out the weight of the solute required for a specified amount of a preparation when required percentage for the preparation is specified.

Q. *Find out the amount of sodium chloride required to prepare 10 L of 0.9% w/v sodium chloride solution.*

Solution:

10 L = 10000 ml

100 ml of solution contain 0.9 g of sodium chloride

Therefore, 10000 ml of solution will contain

$$= \frac{0.9 \times 10000}{100} = 90 \text{ g}$$

Alternative method

$$\text{Required volume of the preparation} \times \frac{\text{given percentage}}{100}$$

$$= \text{Required amount of the solute}$$

or $10000 \text{ ml} \times \dfrac{0.9}{100} = 90$ g of sodium chloride is required

To find the final volume of the liquid preparation when percentage of solute and total amount of solute is provided in the problem.

Q. *Find out how many litres of 0.18% w/v injection can be prepared with 3.6 g of adrenaline bitartrate?*

Solution:

0.18 g of adrenaline bitartrate is present in 100 ml of preparation

Therefore, 3.6 g of adrenaline bitartrate will be present in

$$\frac{100 \times 3.6}{0.18} = 2000 \text{ ml} = 2 \text{ L of solution}$$

Alternative method

3.6 g will be used to prepare 0.18% w/v injection; therefore 3.6 g is directly proportional to 0.18% w/w. Let us consider total amount of the formulation is X g which corresponds to 100% w/w of the preparation.

$$\frac{X}{3.6} = \frac{100}{0.18}$$

$$X = \frac{100 \times 3.6}{0.18} = 2000 \text{ g}$$

If the solvent is water, 2000 g is almost equivalent to 2000 ml. So we have to make up the volume up to 2000 ml (2 litres).

Problems related to percentage volume in volume

To find out the volume of the solute or active ingredient in a specified volume of the preparation with given percentage of the solute or active ingredient.

Q. Find out the volume of chloroform required for preparation 750 ml of 0.25% v/v chloroform water.

Solution:

100 ml of chloroform water contain 0.25 ml of chloroform

Therefore 750 ml of chloroform water will require

$$= \frac{0.25 \times 750}{100} = 1.875 \text{ ml}$$

Alternative method

$$\text{Required volume of the preparation} \times \frac{\text{percentage of solute}}{100}$$

$$= \text{Required amount of the solute}$$

or $750 \times \dfrac{0.25}{100} = 1.875$ ml of chloroform is required

To find out percentage volume in volume of a solute in a liquid preparation for a specified amount of the preparation with given amount of solute.

Q. 500 ml of chlorophenothane application contain 2.5 ml of citronella oil. Find out the percentage of citronella oil in the given preparation.

Solution:

500 ml of chlorophenothane application contain 2.5 ml of citronella oil.

Therefore, 100 ml of chlorophenothane application contains

$$= \frac{2.5 \times 100}{500} = 0.5\% \text{ v/v of citronella oil.}$$

Alternative method

500 ml of the preparation corresponds to 100% v/v of the preparation. Let us consider 2.5 ml of the preparation corresponds to X% v/v of the preparation.

Now,

$$\frac{X}{100} = \frac{2.5}{500}$$

$$X\left(\%\frac{v}{v}\right) = \frac{2.5 \times 100}{500} = 0.5\%\frac{v}{v} \text{ of citronella oil}$$

To find out final volume of the liquid preparation when the volume of solute and percentage of solute in the preparation is provided

Q. What will be the total volume of the preparation if 2.5 ml of datura liquid extract is provided to prepare a 10% v/v preparation?

Solution:

10 ml of datura liquid extract contain in 100 ml of preparation

2.5 ml of datura liquid extract will contain in

$$= \frac{100 \times 2.5}{10} = 25 \text{ ml of preparation}$$

Therefore, final volume of the preparation will be 25 ml.

Alternative method

2.5 ml of datura liquid extract corresponds to 10% v/v of the preparation.

Let X ml of the preparation corresponds to the 100% v/v of the preparation.

$$\frac{X}{2.5} = \frac{100}{100}$$

$$X = \frac{100 \times 2.5}{10} = 25 \text{ ml}$$

25 ml is the total volume of the preparation.

Problems related to percentage weight in weight

To find out the weight of solute in a preparation for specified weight of preparation and given percentage (% w/w) of solute in the preparation

Q. Find out the weight of phosphoric acid required to prepare 250 g of dilute phosphoric acid (11.2% w/w).

Solution:

100 g of dilute phosphoric acid contain 11.2 g of phosphoric acid.

$$250 \text{ g of dilute phosphoric acid contain} = \frac{2.5 \times 11.2}{100} = 28 \text{ g}$$

of phosphoric acid.

Alternative method

$$\text{Required volume of the preparation} \times \frac{\text{given percentage}}{100}$$
$$= \text{Required amount of the solute}$$

$$\text{Required amount of phosphoric acid} = 250 \times \frac{11.2}{100} = 28 \text{ g}$$

Q. Find out the weight of API for preparation 1 L of syrup containing 5% w/w of API having specific gravity of 1.27.

Solution:

1 litre = 1000 ml

Total quantity of syrup in weight = 1000 × 1.27 = 1270 g

Applying the formula, required amount of API

$$= 1270 \times \frac{5}{100} = 63.50 \text{ g}$$

To find out the percentage strength of solute in a formulation when weight of active ingredient and weight of the preparation are provided.

Q. 15 g of API is mixed with other ingredients to prepare 120 g of a formulation. What is the percentage strength of API in the formulation?

Solution:

120 g of the formulation contain 15 g of API

Therefore, 100 g of the formulation contain $= \dfrac{100 \times 15}{120}$

= 12.5 g of API

Therefore, percentage strength of API in the formulation = 12.5% w/w

Alternative method

120 g of the formulation corresponds to 100% w/w of the formulation. Let us consider, 15 g of API corresponds to X% w/w of the formulation.

$$\frac{X}{100} = \frac{15}{120}$$
$$X = \frac{15 \times 100}{120} = 12.5\% \text{ w/w of API}$$

Q. 77 g of sugar is dissolved in water to make the volume up to 100 ml. If the specific gravity of the syrup is 1.149, what is the percentage strength (% w/w) of sugar in the syrup?

Solution:

The weight of 100 ml of syrup = 100 × 1.149 = 114.9 g

Percentage strength of sugar $= \dfrac{77 \times 100}{114.9} = 67.01\%$ w/w

Q. If 4 g of dextrose is dissolved in 76 ml of water, what will be the percentage strength of dextrose in the formulation?

Solution:

The weight of 76 ml of water is almost equivalent to 76 g of water. Therefore, total weight of the formulation = 76 + 4 = 80 g.

Percentage strength of dextrose $= \dfrac{4 \times 100}{80} = 5\%$ w/w

To find out the total weight of the formulation when percentage strength and weight of active pharmaceutical ingredient is provided.

Q. Find out the total amount of liquefied phenol (80% w/w) can be prepared with 200 g of phenol.

Solution:

80 g of phenol gives 100 g of liquefied phenol

Therefore, 200 g of phenol will give

$$= \frac{100 \times 200}{80} = 250 \text{ g of liquefied phenol}$$

Alternative method

200 g of the formulation is equivalent to 80% w/w of the formulation. Let us consider X g of the formulation will be equivalent to 100% w/w of the formulation.

$$\frac{X}{200} = \frac{100}{80}$$

$$X = \frac{100 \times 200}{80} = 250 \text{ g}$$

Therefore, the total weight of the formulation is 250 g.

PROBLEMS

1. 350 ml of solution contains 250 mg of a drug. Calculate the percentage strength and ratio strength of the solution?

2. Calamine lotion contains 15% w/v calamine. Find out how much amount of calamine should be used to formulate 250 ml of calamine lotion?

3. How many millilitres of ammoniated camphor liniment can be prepared from 3 g of camphor if percentage strength of the liniment is 12.5% w/v?

4. Chloroform spirit contains 0.5% v/v chloroform. How many millilitres of chloroform spirit can be prepared using 14.9 g of chloroform?

5. Find out the total volume of the final preparation if 12 ml of anise oil should be used to prepare 0.3% v/v solution?

6. How many grams of simple ointment can be prepared from 25 g of wool fat if its percentage strength is 5% w/v?

7. A formulation was prepared by mixing 17 g of drug with 153 g of ointment base. What is the percentage strength of the drug in the formulation?

8. Find out the percentage strength of each ingredient in the given formulation. Also find out the quantity of each ingredient required to prepare 50 ml of the formulation.

Ingredients	Official formula
Terpin hydrate	50 g
Orange oil	0.2 ml
Glycerin	400 ml
Alcohol	425 ml
Syrup	100 ml
Purified water, sufficient quantity to make up to 1000 ml	

9. 40 ml of turpentine liniment contain 26 ml of turpentine oil. What is the percentage strength of turpentine oil?

10. 100 g of a syrup formulation contain 5 mg of active pharmaceutical excipient. If the specific gravity of the syrup is 1.135, what is the percentage strength (% w/v) of the drug?

11. How many grams of an active pharmaceutical excipient should be dissolved in 500 ml water to prepare 10% w/w solution?

12. What is the percentage strength of the solution prepared by dissolving 52 g of sulphuric acid in 448 ml of water?

13. The percentage strength of a preservative in a formulation is 0.0025% w/v. If the volume of the solution is 50 ml, find out how many micrograms of the preservative present in the formulation.

14. A physician prescribes 50 mg of an active pharmaceutical ingredient in normal saline solution to a patient. How many millilitres of 1% w/v normal saline solution of the drug should be supplied to patient?

15. 5 ml of flavoring agent was added to a 10 litres batch of syrup. Find out the percentage strength of the flavoring agent.

16. How many grams of dextrose should be required to prepare 750 ml of 5% w/v solution of dextrose?

4 Calculation Based on Parts Per Notation

CALCULATION BASED ON PARTS PER NOTATION

Parts per notation are used to express the values of dimensionless fractions. It is used to describe very small values. No units of measurement are associated with them. Most commonly used parts per notation is parts per million (ppm). Apart from these parts per billion (ppb), parts per trillion (ppt) are used but there meanings are language dependent. Such as, ppt is sometimes read as parts per thousand. When parts per notation are used, one should state dimensionless quantity whose value is being stated.

Table 4.1 Notation and coefficient

Name	Notation	Coefficient
Parts per hundredhundred (percent)	%	10^{-2}
Parts per million	ppm	10^{-6}
Parts per billion	ppb	10^{-9}
Parts per trillion	ppt	10^{-12}

Parts per notation are commonly used to express dilute solution. Parts per notation may refer to volume fraction, mass fraction or mole fraction. So, it is necessary to state the quantity involved. Parts per notation are used for expression of value of dimensionless quantities.

ppmw – It is used to denote ppm when ppm is determined in terms of weight of solute and solution.

ppmv – It is used to denote ppm when ppm is determined in terms of volume of solute and solution.

Mathematical formula for calculation of parts per million

$$C_{ppm} = 10^6 \times \frac{m_{solute}}{m_{solvent} + m_{solute}}$$

C_{ppm} – Concentration of solute in parts per million

m_{solute} – Mass of the solute

$m_{solution}$ – Mass of solvent

As $m_{solute} \ll m_{solvent}$, we can neglect the mass of solute.

$$C_{ppm} = 10^6 \times \frac{m_{solute}}{m_{solvent}}$$

The above equation refers to mass fraction. Similar calculation can be done for volume fraction and mole fraction.

Conversion of ppm to decimal fraction

$$P_d = \frac{P_{ppm}}{10^6}$$

P_d – Parts of solute in decimal fraction

P_{ppm} – Parts of solute in ppm

Conversion of ppm to percent

$$C(\%) = \frac{P_{ppm}}{10^4}$$

$C(\%)$ – Percentage concentration of solute

Conversion of milligram per litre to C_{ppm}

$$C_{ppm} = \frac{C_{(mg/L)}}{\rho_{g/ml}}$$

$C_{(mg/L)}$ – Concentration of the solute (mg/L)

$\rho(kg/m^3)$ – Density of solution in kilogram per cubic metre

Conversion of gram per litre to C_{ppm}

$$C_{ppm} = 1000 \times \frac{C_{(g/L)}}{\rho_{g/ml}}$$

$C_{(g/L)}$ – Concentration of solute in gram per litre

Conversion of mole per litre to C_{ppm}

$$C_{ppm} = 1000 \times \frac{C_{mol/L} \times M}{\rho_{g/ml}}$$

$C_{mol/L}$ – Concentration of solute in mole per litre
M – Molar mass of the solute

Conversion of C_{ppm} into C_{ppb}

$$C_{ppb} = \frac{C_{ppm}}{1000}$$

C_{ppb} – Concentration of solute in parts per billion

SOLVED PROBLEMS

1. Express 0.001% v/v solution in ppm.
   Solution:

   $$C_{ppm} = 0.001 \times 10^4 = 10 \text{ ppm}$$

2. How many millilitres of chloroform are required to prepare 1000 ml, 2500 ppm chloroform water?
   Solution:

   $$C_{ppm} = 10^6 \times \frac{\text{Volume of solute (ml)}}{\text{Volume of solution (ml)}}$$

   $$\text{Volume of chloroform} = \frac{2500 \times 1000}{10^6} = 250 \text{ ppm}$$

3. 1000 ml of piperazine citrate elixir contains 0.25 ml of orange oil. Express the concentration of orange oil in ppm.
   Solution:

   $$C_{ppm} = \frac{0.25}{1000} \times 10^6 = 250 \text{ ppm}$$

   250 ppm of orange oil present in piperazine citrate elixir.

PROBLEMS

1. Express 1 ppm into percentage.
2. Express 1 ppm into decimal fraction.
3. The concentration of a drug in a solution is 10 ppm. Express the concentration of drug in ppb.
4. Density of a solution is 1 g/ml. The concentration of the drug in the solution is 2000 ppm. Find out the concentration of the drug in mg/L.
5. A stock solution contains 10 mg of drug per 100 ml solution. From this stock solution, 1 ml solution was diluted upto 10 ml. Find out the concentration of drug in ppm. Given that 1ml of solution weighs 1 g.
6. How will you prepare calcium standard solution (10 ppm Ca) using dried calcium carbonate?
7. How will you prepare chlorine standard solution (5 ppm Cl) using sodium chloride?
8. How will you prepare ammonium standard solution (1 ppm NH_4) using 0.0741% w/v solution?
9. How will you prepare nitrate standard solution (100 ppm NO_3, 2 ppm NO_3) using potassium nitrate?
10. Silver standard solution (5 ppm Ag) is prepared by diluting 1 volume of a stock solution to 100 volumes with water. Find out the percentage strength (% w/v) of silver nitrate in the stock solution?
11. 0.4 g of lead nitrate is dissolved in water containing 2 ml nitric acid and volume is made upto 100 ml with water. How will you prepare lead standard solution containing 100 ppm Pb, 20 ppm Pb, 2 ppm Pb and 1 ppm Pb?

Conversion of Milliequivalent and Milliosmolar Value

5

Equivalent weight is the mass of one equivalent equal to the mass of a given substance, which will

i. Supply or react with one mole of electrons in a redox reaction

ii. Supply or react with one mole of protons in an acid base reaction

iii. Combine or displace directly or indirectly with 1.008 parts by mass of hydrogen or 8 parts by mass of oxygen or 35.5 parts by mass of chlorine.

Equivalent weight can be found out by dividing the atomic weight by the usual valence or dividing the molecular weight by the total valence of positive or negative radical.

One milliequivalent is 1/1000 of an equivalent. Therefore, 1 equivalent weight is 1000 milliequivalent weight. It is commonly used for expression concentration of electrolyte in solution.

Osmole is a unit of measurement, which defines the number of moles of solute in a solution that contribute to the osmotic pressure of the solution. Let us consider 1 mole of KCl is dissolved in water and volume is made up to 1000 ml. Concentration of KCl can be expressed as 1 mole/L but it will give a concentration of 2 osmol/L in respect of osmolarity. In solution, one mole of potassium chloride is divided into two osmoles because formation of one mole of K^+ and one mole of Cl^- from KCl molecule due to ionization.

A milliosmole is $1/1000$ of an osmole. It is one of the units most frequently used for preparation of electrolyte solution in water.

Conversion of percentage weight per volume to milliequivalent per unit volume.

Q. Convert 0.9% w/v solution of sodium chloride into milliequivalents (mEq) of sodium chloride per unit ml.

Solution:

Molecular weight of sodium chloride = 58.5

Equivalent weight of sodium chloride = 58.5

$$1 \text{ mEq of sodium chloride} = 58.5 \times \frac{1}{1000} = 0.0585 \text{ g}$$

0.9 % w/v of sodium chloride = 0.9 g of sodium chloride per 100 ml

= 0.009 g of sodium chloride per ml

$$0.9 \% \text{ w/v of sodium chloride solution} = \frac{0.009}{0.0585}$$

= 0.1538 mEq per ml

or it can be expressed as 153.8 mEq of sodium chloride per litre.

Conversion of milligrams percent to milliequivalents per litre

Q. Express the concentration of a solution contains 10 mg % of Mg^{+2} ions in mEq per litre.

Solution:

Atomic weight of magnesium = 24

$$\text{Equivalent weight of } Mg^{+2} = \frac{24}{2} = 12$$

10 mg % of Mg^{2+} = 10 mg of Mg^{2+} per 100 ml of solution

= 100 mg of Mg^{2+} per 1000 ml of solution

$$10 \text{ mg \% of } Mg^{+2} \text{ ion} = \frac{100}{12} = 8.33 \text{ mEq of Mg ion per litre}$$

Conversion of milliequivalent per unit volume to percentage weight per volume.

Q. What is the percentage concentration (% w/v) of a solution containing 154 mEq of sodium chloride per litre?

Solution:

Molecular weight of NaCl = 58.5

Equivalent weight of NaCl = 58.5

$$1 \text{ milliequivalent of NaCl} = \frac{1}{1000} \times 58.5 = 0.0585 \text{ g}$$

1000 ml of solution contain = 9.009 g of NaCl

$$100 \text{ ml of solution will contain} = \frac{9.009}{1000} \times 100 = 0.9009 \text{ g}$$

of NaCl

Therefore, percentage strength of the given solution is 0.9009 % w/v.

Conversion of milliequivalent per unit volume to milligrams per ml

Q. Find out the concentration in terms of mg per ml of a solution 277.78 milliequivalents of dextrose per litre of the formulation.

Solution:

Molecular weight of anhydrous dextrose = 180

Equivalent weight of anhydrous dextrose = 180

$$1 \text{ milliequivalent of dextrose} = \frac{1}{1000} \times 180 = 0.180 \text{ g}$$

$$= \frac{180}{1} \times 277.8 = 50004 \text{ g/L}$$

$$= 50.004 \text{ mg per ml}$$

To find out the amount of substance or volume of its solution for a specific concentration for to supply a specific amount milliequivalent level to a patient.

Q. How many millilitres of isotonic sodium chloride are required to provide 90 mEq of sodium chloride to a patient?

Solution:

We know that the concentration of isotonic solution is 0.9 % w/v. Therefore, 1000 ml of 0.9 % w/v sodium chloride solution contain 9 g of sodium chloride.

Molecular weight of sodium chloride = 58.5

Equivalent weight of sodium chloride = 58.5

98 mEq of sodium chloride = 90 × 0.0585 = 5.265 g

Therefore, 9 g of sodium chloride is present in 1000 ml of solution.

5.265 g of sodium chloride is present in

$$= \frac{5.265}{9} \times 1000 = 585 \text{ ml of solution}$$

Q. The weight of a patient is 70 kg. The patient needs 2.4 mEq of sodium chloride per kilogram of body weight. How many millilitres of isotonic sodium chloride solution are required to supply desired milliequivalents of sodium chloride?

Solution:

It is given that

1. Weight of patient = 70 kg
2. Specific amount of milliequivalent to be supply = 2.4 mEq of sodium chloride

Therefore, total milliequivalents to be supply to the patient = 70 × 2.4 = 168 mEq of sodium chloride

1 mEq of sodium chloride = 0.0585 g

168 mEq of sodium chloride = 168 × 0.0585 = 9.828 g of sodium chloride

9 g sodium chloride contain in 1000 ml of solution

9.828 g sodium chloride contain in $= \dfrac{9.828 \times 1000}{9} = 1092 \text{ ml}$

Therefore, 1092 ml of sodium chloride is required to supply to the patient.

To find out the milliequivalent of constituent ion in a specified amount substance

Q. Find out the milliequivalent of sodium ions (Na⁺) present in 5 g of ampicillin sodium.

Solution:

Atomic weight of Na⁺ = 23

Atomic weight of sodium = 23

1 milliequivalent of Na⁺ = 23 mg

371 mg of ampicillin sodium contain = 23 mg of Na⁺

5000 mg of ampicillin sodium contain $= \dfrac{23 \times 5000}{371} = 309.97 \text{ mg}$

Required milliequivalent of sodium ion (Na^+) = $\dfrac{309.97}{23}$

= 13.477 mEq of sodium ion (Na^+)

To find out the amount of a substance required to prepare a solution of specific milliequivalent for specified volume

Q. Find out the amount of sodium bicarbonate required to prepare 100 ml of a solution containing 1 mEq per ml.

Solution:

Molecular weight of sodium bicarbonate = 84

Equivalent weight of sodium bicarbonate = 84

100 ml of solution contain = 100 mEq of sodium bicarbonate

100 mEq of sodium bicarbonate = 100 × 84 = 8400 mg = 8.4 g of sodium bicarbonate

8.4 g of sodium bicarbonate is required to prepare 100 ml of 1 mEq solution of sodium bicarbonate.

Conversion of percentage weight per volume to milliosmols per litre

Q. Convert the concentration of 1 % w/v solution of potassium chloride to milliosmols per litre.

Solution:

Molecular weight of KCl = 74.5

1 millimol of KCl = 2 milliosmols of KCl (K^+ and Cl^-)

= 74.5 mg

100 ml of potassium chloride solution contain = 1 g of potassium chloride

1000 ml of potassium chloride solution will contain

$= \dfrac{1000 \times 1}{100}$ = 10 g of potassium chloride

10 g of potassium chloride = 10000 mg of potassium chloride

74.5 mg of potassium chloride = 2 milliosmols

$10000 \text{ mg of potassium chloride} = \dfrac{10000}{74.5} \times 2 = 268.46 \text{ mOsm/L}$

Therefore, 1% w/v solution of potassium chloride is equivalent to 268.46 milliosmols per litre.

Q. Convert 10% w/v dextrose solution into milliosmols per litre.
Solution:

Molecular weight of dextrose = 180

1 millimol of dextrose = 1 milliosmol of dextrose = 180 mg of dextrose

10 % w/v solution of dextrose contain 10 g of dextrose per 100 ml of the solution

Therefore, 1000 ml of the solution contain 100 g or 100000 mg dextrose.

Required milliosmols per litre = $\dfrac{100000}{180}$ = 555.55 mOsm/L

Q. Convert 20 mg.% of Ca^{+2} ions into milliosmols per litre.
Solution:

Atomic weight of Ca^{+2} = 40

1 millimol = 1 milliosmol = 40 mg

It is given that

100 ml of solution contain 20 mg of Ca^{+2} ions

1000 ml of solution contain = $\dfrac{20 \times 1000}{100}$ = 200 mg of Ca^{+2}

Required milliosmol per litre = $\dfrac{200}{40}$ = 5 mEq per litre

Conversion of milliosmols per litre to percentage weight per volume.

Q. Convert 308 mOsm per litre of sodium chloride solution into percentage weight per volume?
Solution:

Molecular weight of sodium chloride = 58.5

1 millimol = 2 milliosmol = 58.5 mg

2 milliosmol of sodium chloride = 58.5 mg sodium chloride

308 milliosmol of sodium chloride = $\dfrac{58.5 \times 308}{2}$ = 9009 mg

= 9.009 g sodium chloride

Percentage concentration of sodium chloride (% w/v)

= $\dfrac{9.009}{1000} \times 100$ = 0.9009 % w/v

PROBLEMS

1. Calculate milliequivalents (mEq) of a 10% w/v potassium chloride solution.
2. Calculate milliequivalents (mEq) of 0.26% w/v sodium chloride solution.
3. Calculate milliequivalents (mEq) of 14.7% w/v calcium chloride dihydrate solution.
4. Calculate milliequivalents (mEq) of 5 mg % of sodium ion.
5. Calculate milliequivalents (mEq) of 2 mg % of calcium ions.
6. What is the percentage concentration of a solution containing 0.154 mEq of sodium chloride per ml?
7. What is the milligrams percent of a solution containing 5 mEq of potassium ion per litre?
8. What is the milligrams percent of a solution containing 2 mEq of magnesium ion per litre?
9. How many grams of sodium chloride should be used to prepare 5 litres of 0.154 mEq per ml?
10. A patient needs 2 mEq of sodium/kg. If the body weight of the person is 70 kg, how many millilitres of 0.9% w/v sodium chloride should be supplied to patient?
11. A solution contains 513 mEq of sodium chloride per litre. How many grams of sodium chloride present in 50 ml of the solution?
12. A solution contains 4 mEq/L of K^+. Find out how many grams of potassium chloride should be used to obtain 100 ml of solution?
13. A child needs 10 mEq of potassium per day. How many milligrams of potassium is needed by the child?
14. How will you prepare 1 litre solution of 77 mEq sodium chloride?
15. What is the concentration of a 0.18% w/v sodium chloride solution in terms of milliequivalents?
16. How many millilitres of 0.5% w/v sodium chloride solution should be supplied to provide 90 mEq of sodium chloride?

17. Calculate milliequivalents sodium ions (Na^+) present in 100 mg of diclofenac sodium.

18. How many milliequivalents of potassium present in 500 mg of amoxicillin potassium?

19. 2.6 g of sodium chloride present in 1 litre of solution. Calculate milliosmols per litre considering complete dissociation of sodium chloride.

6

Ratio Strength

MATHEMATICAL PROBLEMS RELATED TO RATIO STRENGTH OF PHARMACEUTICAL PRODUCT

Ratio strength is frequently used in pharmaceutical formulation to designate concentration. 1:100 which is a ratio strength can be interpreted for different formulation such as:

For solids in solids: 1 g of constituent per 100 g of the formulation

For liquids in liquids: 1 ml of constituent per 100 ml of the formulation

For solids in liquids: 1 g of constituent per 100 ml of the formulation

To find percentage strength for the given ratio strength

Q. Convert 1:2000 into percentage strength.

Solution:

We know that 2000 parts is equivalent to 100% of formulation. Let us consider 1 part is equivalent to x% of the formulation.

$$\frac{x}{100} = \frac{1}{2000}$$

$$x = \frac{100}{2000} = 0.05\ \%$$

Alternative method

2000 parts represent = 100 %

$$1 \text{ part represents } \frac{100 \times 1}{2000} = 0.05\%$$

To find out ratio strength for given percentage strength

Q. Convert 0.5% into ratio strength.

Solution:

For the given problem, 0.5% is equal to 1 part.

Let us consider X parts represent 100%.

$$\frac{X}{1} = \frac{100}{0.5}$$

$$X = \frac{100 \times 1}{0.5} = 200 \text{ parts}$$

Ratio strength for 0.5% is 1:200.

Formulation Problems

Q. How many of millilitres of hyoscyamus liquids extract are required to prepare 5 litres of a 1:10 Hyoscyamus tincture?

Solution:

5 litres = 5000 ml

Let x ml of hyoscyamus liquids extract is required to prepare 5000 ml of 1:10 hyoscyamus tincture. It is given that 1 ml Hyoscyamus liquids extract contain in 10 ml of tincture.

$$\frac{X}{1} = \frac{5000}{10}$$

$$X = \frac{5000 \times 1}{10} = 500 \text{ ml}$$

Alternative method

10 ml of tincture contain 1 ml of hyoscyamus liquid extract

Therefore, 5000 ml tincture contain

$$= \frac{1 \times 5000}{10} = 500 \text{ ml of hyoscyamus liquid extract}$$

Or

Required amount of product × ratio strength = Required amount of constituent

$$= \frac{1 \times 5000}{10} = 500 \text{ ml of hyoscyamus liquid extract is required}$$

Q. A dextrose preparation contains 5 g of dextrose in 100 ml of water. Find out the ratio strength for the formulation.

Solution:

5 g of dextrose contain in 100 ml of water

1 g of dextrose contain in $\dfrac{100 \times 1}{5} = 20$ ml of water

Ratio strength = 1:20

Q. 5 mg of active pharmaceutical ingredient contain in 500 ml of plant extract. Find out the ratio strength.

Solution:

5 mg of API = $\dfrac{5}{1000} = 0.005$ g

0.005 g of API is present in 500 ml of plant extract

1 g of API contain in = $\dfrac{1 \times 500}{0.005} = 100000$

Ratio strength = 1:100000

Alternative method

Let X ml of plant extract contains 1 g of active pharmaceutical ingredient.

$$\frac{X}{500} = \frac{1}{0.005}$$

$$X = \frac{500}{0.005} = 100000$$

Ratio strength = 1:100000

Q. How many milligrams of drug are required to prepare 350 ml of a 1:20000 solution?

Solution:

20000 ml of the solution contain 1 g of drug.

350 ml of the solution contain = $\dfrac{350 \times 1}{2000} = 0.0175$ g = 17.5 mg of drug

PROBLEMS

Q. Convert 1:5000 into percentage strength.

Q. Convert 1% into ratio strength.

Q. How many millilitres of a drug should be used to formulate 100 ml of 1:10 drug solution?

Q. A sodium chloride solution contains 100 mg of sodium chloride per 100 ml of the solution. Find out the ratio strength of the solution.

Q. An injection contains 0.1% w/v of drug A and 1:50000 (w/v) of drug B. Find out the ratio strength of drug A and percentage strength of drug B in the injection.

Q. A stock solution contains 5% w/v of a drug. How will you prepare 1:10000 (w/v) solution from the stock solution?

Q. A vial contains 10 ml of a drug solution. The ratio strength of drug in the solution is 1:5000. How much amount of drug present in the vial?

Q. Ratio strength of a stock solution if a drug is 1:100 (w/v). How will prepare you prepare 0.001% w/v solution from the stock solution?

Q. An eye drop contains 1:5000 (w/v) of benzalkonium chloride. How much amount of benzalkonium chloride is required to prepare one US gallon of eye drop formulation?

7 Enlarging and Reducing a Pharmaceutical Formula

MATHEMATICAL APPROACH TO FIND OUT THE QUANTITIES OF INGREDIENTS FOR ENLARGING OR REDUCING A FORMULA FOR REQUIRED AMOUNT OF THE FORMULATION

Step I: At first, we have to find out the total amount of the formulation given in the formula (X).

Step II: Find out the total amount to be produced during preparation (Y).

Step III: Divide Y by X, it will give the multiplication factor for further calculation.

$$\text{Multiplication factor} = \frac{Y}{X}$$

Step IV: Multiply the quantity of each ingredient given in the formula with this multiplication factor, you will get the required quantity of the ingredient for the specified total amount.

Q. Find out the quantities of each ingredient required to prepare 750 ml of benzyl benzoate lotion.

Name of the Ingredient	Quantity
Benzyl benzoate	250 ml
Triethanolamine	5 g
Oleic acid	20 g
Purified Water, make up to	1000 ml

Solution:

Step I: Total amount given in the formula = 1000 ml

Step II: Total amount of the preparation to be prepared = 750 ml

Step III: Multiplication factor $\dfrac{750}{1000}$ = 0.75

Step IV: Required amount of each ingredient,

Benzyl benzoate = 250 × 0.75 = 187.50 ml

Triethanolamine = 5 × 0.75 = 3.75 g

Oleic acid = 20 × 0.75 = 15 g

Purified water, make up to 750 ml.

So, we have to add 187.50 ml of benzyl benzoate, 3.75 g of Triethanolamine, 15 g of oleic acid to the prepare the formulation for the specified total amount. This involves reducing a given formula as per need.

Q. *Find out the quantities of each ingredient required to prepare 1.5 L of piperazine citrate elixir.*

Ingredients	Official Formula
Piperazine citrate	180 g
Chloroform spirit	5 ml
Glycerin	100 ml
Orange oil	0.25 ml
Syrup	500 ml
Purified water, sufficient to produce 1000 ml	

Solution:

Step I: Total amount given in the formula = 1000 ml

Step II: The required amount to be prepared = 1.5 L = 1500 ml

Step III: Multiplication factor = $\dfrac{1500}{1000}$ = 1.5

Step IV: Required amount of each ingredient,

Piperazine citrate = 1.5 × 180 = 270 g

Chloroform spirit = 5 × 1.5 = 7.5 ml

Glycerin = 100 × 1.5 = 150 ml

Orange oil = 0.25 × 1.5 = 0.375 ml

Syrup = 500 × 1.5 = 750 ml

Purified water, make up to 1500 ml.

The above calculation involves the enlargement of the formula.

Finding out the quantities of ingredients for enlarging or reducing a formula for required amount of the formulation using proportional parts. When the formula specifies number of parts for each ingredient

Q. Find out the quantities of each ingredient given in the formula to prepare 50 g paraffin ointment.

Ingredients	Formula
White beeswax	2 parts
Hard paraffin	3 parts
Cetostearyl alcohol	5 parts
White soft paraffin or yellow soft paraffin	90 parts

Solution:

Total number of parts by weight = 100

Let consider required amount of white beeswax, hard paraffin, cetostearyl alcohol and white soft paraffin are 2X, 3X, 5X, 90X respectively.

Now, we have

$$2X + 3X + 5X + 90X = 50$$

$$100X = 50$$

$$X = \frac{50}{100} = 0.5$$

So, required amount of the following ingredients are:

White beeswax = 2 × 0.5 = 1 g

Hard paraffin = 3 × 0.5 = 1.5 g

Cetostearyl alcohol = 5 × 0.5 = 2.5 g

White soft paraffin = 90 × 0.5 = 45 g

When all the ingredients are measured by weight alone or volume alone, one can express all the weights (or all volumes) in parts provided that they have the common denomination.

Q. Find out the quantity of each ingredient required to prepare 350 g of rhubarb compound powder.

Ingredients	Formula
Rhubarb, finely powdered	20 g
Light magnesium carbonate	26 g
Heavy magnesium carbonate	26 g
Ginger, finely powdered	8 g

Solution:

First, consider the number of grams of ingredients as number of parts. Therefore, the number of parts of rhubarb, finely powdered in the given formula is 20 parts.

Let us consider the required quantities of each ingredient are 20X, 26X, 26X and 8X.

Now, we have

$$20X + 26 + 26X + 8X = 350$$

$$X = \frac{350}{80} = 4.375$$

Qauntity of rhubarb, finely powdered required = 20 × 4.375 = 87.5 g

Quantity of magnesium carbonate required = 26 × 4.375 = 113.75 g

Quantity of heavy magnesium carbonate required = 26 × 4.375 = 113.75 g

Quantity of ginger, finely powdered required = 8 × 4.375 = 35 g

PROBLEMS

1. Calculate the amount of each ingredient to be used to formulate 100 g of formulation given below.

Ingredients	Official Formula
Acetylsalicylic acid	0.3 g
Citric acid	0.03 g
Calcium carbonate	0.1 g
Saccharin sodium	3 mg

2. Calculate the amount of each ingredient to be used to formulate 10 pounds of formulation. How many tablet can be formulated from 10 pounds of formulation if each tablet contains

Ingredients	Official Formula
Acetylsalicylic acid	0.25 g
Phenacetin	0.25 g
Codeine phosphate	8 mg

3. How will you dispense 50 ml of Ipecacuanha tincture for the given formula?

Ingredients	Official Formula
Ipecacuanha liquid extract	100 ml
Dilute acetic acid	16.5 ml
Alcohol (90% v/v)	210 ml
Glycerin	200 ml
Purified water, sufficient to produce	1000 ml

4. How will you prepare 100 g of wool alcohols ointment from the following formula?

Ingredients	Official Formula
Wool alcohols	60 parts
Hard paraffin	240 parts
White soft paraffin or yellow soft paraffin	100 parts
Liquid paraffin	600 parts

5. How will you prepare 1 US gallon of compound sodium chloride solution from the following formula?

Ingredients	Official Formula
Sodium chloride	8.6 g
Potassium chloride	0.30 g
Calcium chloride hydrated	0.33 g
Purified water, recently boiled, sufficient quantity to produce	1000 ml

6. How will you prepare 0.1 pounds of zinc undecylenate ointment from the following formula?

Ingredients	Official Formula
Zinc undecylenate	200 parts
Undecylenic ointment	50 parts
Emulsifying ointment	750 parts

7. 5000 tablets were prepared from a batch of the given formula without any loss. How many grams of each ingredient were used for the batch?

Ingredients	Official Formula
Calcium gluconate	0.5 g
Sucrose	1.0 g
Mentha oil	0.0015 ml

8

Alligation Method

Alligation is a calculation technique which is used to find out the proportions of substances of different strengths must be mixed in order to get a mixture of required strength. The word alligation comes from Latin word *alligatio* which means the act of attaching. The proportion of different substances is found out to get an intermediate strength, calculation can be done to find out exact amounts of different substances required to produce a required amount of the desired substance.

There are two types of alligation method.

1. Alligation alternate is a technique by which one can find out the parts or amount of same formulation of different percentage strength or base is required to prepare the formulation of specific percentage strength.

2. Alligation medial is the technique by which one can find out percentage strength of a mixture formulation when it is prepared from formulations of the same substance of different percentage strength.

STEPS INVOLVED IN ALLIGATION

Alternative method

It basically involves three columns.

1. All the starting materials are taken in 1st column (left side) and the substances are placed in order of concentration from higher to lower.

2. Desired concentration is placed in the middle column at the middle position.

3. Cross subtraction of middle column from 1st column is done which gives the parts of different concentration required to prepare desired concentration. This constitutes the third column.

Mathematical representation

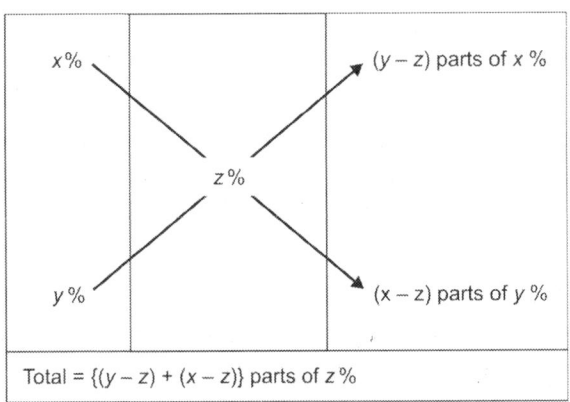

While finding out the parts, negative sign is not considered.

Algebraic method

Let us consider $(y - z) = a$ and $(x - z) = b$

From the given data, we can have

$$ax + by = z(a + b)$$
$$ax + by = za + zb$$
$$\frac{a}{b} = \frac{z - y}{x - z}$$

So using the above equation, we can directly find out required parts of two concentrations to prepare a formulation of specific concentration.

PROBLEMS

To solve problems by Alligation alternate technique

1. Strengths of two alcohol solutions are 15% v/v and 90% v/v. Find out the proportion of the two alcohol solutions to get

an intermediate strength of 40% v/v. How much amount of both the alcohol solutions is required to produce 250 ml of 40% v/v alcohol solution?

Solution: By alligation method:

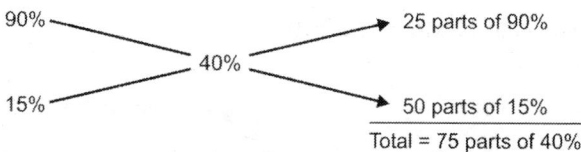

Now, required amount of both alcohol solutions are

Volume of 90% v/v alcohol required = $\dfrac{25}{75} \times 250 = 83.33$ ml

Volume of 15% v/v alcohol required = $\dfrac{50}{75} \times 25\ 0 = 166.67$ ml

2. How many grams of cream containing 2% w/w of active pharmaceutical excipient should be mixed with 20 grams of cream containing 1% w/w of active pharmaceutical ingredient in order to get cream containing 1.5% w/w of active pharmaceutical ingredient?

Solution: By alligation method,

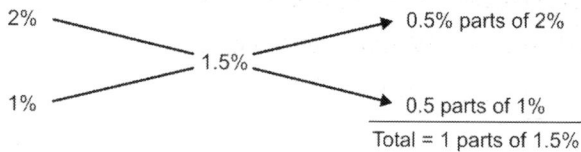

So, 0.5 part of 1% is equal to 20 g.

Weight of 2% w/w cream required

$= \dfrac{0.5 \text{ part of } 2\% \text{ w/w}}{0.5 \text{ part of } 1\% \text{ w/w}} \times 20 \text{ g of } 1\% \text{ w/w cream}$

$= 20 \text{ g of } 2\% \text{ w/w cream}$

3. A gel contains 2% w/w of active pharmaceutical ingredient. Find out the amount of pure drug and 2% w/w gel required to prepare 100 g of a gel containing 10% w/w of active pharmaceutical ingredient.

Solution: By alligation method:

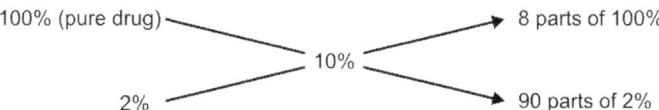

Amount of pure drug required = $\dfrac{8}{98}$ × 100 = 8.16 g

Amount of 2% w/w gel required = $\dfrac{90}{98}$ × 100 = 91.84 g

MIXING OF MULTIPLE COMPOSITIONS

4. In what proportion should 30% w/v, 15% w/v and 2.5% w/v dextrose solution should be mixed to prepare a 5% w/v dextrose solution?

Solution:

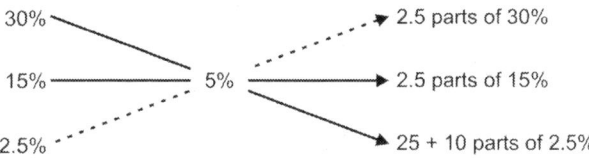

Ratio of mixing: 2.5:2.5:35

5. In what proportion, 25% w/w, 20% w/w, 7% w/w and 5% w/w zinc oxide ointments should be mixed to get 10% w/w ointment?

Solution: In this case, we have to pair one of the weaker lots with one of the stronger lots. Similarly pairing is done for the remaining weaker and stronger lot. As we can pair 25% w/w lot either with 7% w/w lot or 5% w/w lot, so two ways of pairing is possible.

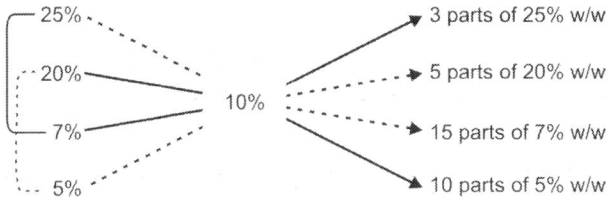

Ratio of mixing: 3:5:15:10

or

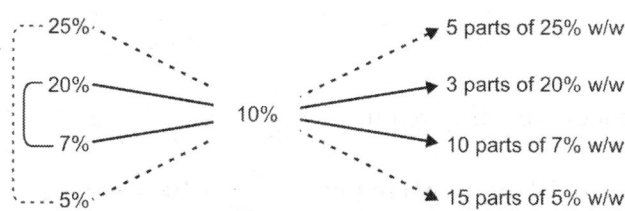

Ratio of mixing: 5:3:10:15

6. How many grams of 3.5% w/w of lidocaine cream should be mixed with 450 gm of 0.5% w/w lidocaine to produce 1% w/w lidocaine cream?

Solution:

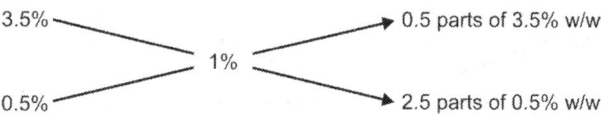

Ratio of mixing: 0.5:2.5 or 1:5

So, one part of 3.5% w/w cream should be mixed with five parts 0.5% w/w cream to produce 1% w/w lidocaine cream. As five parts of 0.5% w/w lidocaine cream is equal 450 g for the given problem, so we can find out amount of 3.5% w/w lidocaine cream by the following formula

$$\frac{\text{Amount of 3.5\% w/w lidocaine cream}}{\text{Amount of 0.5\% w/w lidocaine cream}} = \frac{\text{Parts of 3.5\% w/w}}{\text{Parts of 0.5\% w/w}}$$

$$\text{Amount of 3.5\% w/w lidocaine cream} = \frac{0.5 \times 450}{2.5} = 100 \text{ g}$$

7. How many grams of base should be added to 5% w/w fluconazole cream to prepare 100 g of 1% w/w cream?

Solution:

Let the amount base required to prepare 1% w/w cream is X g.

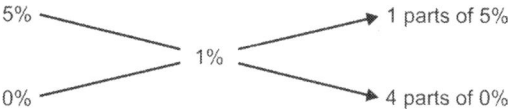

Total parts $= 1 + 4 = 5$ parts

Amount of base is required $= \dfrac{4}{5} \times 100 = 80$ g

To problems by Alligation medial method

Q. Find out the percentage strength of drug in a cream prepared by mixing 50 g of 10% w/w cream, 25 g of 7.5% w/w cream, 10 g of 1% w/w cream.

Solution:

Final percentage strength of mixture

$$= \frac{50 \times 10 + 25 \times 7.5 + 10 \times 1}{85} = \frac{697.5}{85} = 8.2059 \% \, \text{w/w}$$

Q. Find out the percentage strength of drug in a gel prepared by mixing 350 g of 25% w/w gel, 100 g of 10% w/w gel, 250 g of 5% w/w gel and 300 g of gel base.

Solution:

Final percentage strength of gel

$$= \frac{350 \times 25 + 100 \times 10 + 250 \times 5 + 300 \times 0}{350 + 100 + 250 + 300}$$

$$= \frac{11000}{1000} = 11 \% \, \text{w/w}$$

PROBLEMS

1. How much volume of 0.5% w/v drug solution and 1.5% w/v drug solution should be mixed in order to get 100 ml of 1% w/v drug solution?

2. Find out the amount of ointment containing 2% w/w of API and ointment containing 10% w/w of API required to produce 500 g of an ointment containing 5% w/w of API?

3. Prepare 1 kg of ointment containing 2% w/w of API from pure drug and ointment containing 0.5% w/w of API.

4. Prepare a sugar solution coating 10% w/v sugar from sugar solutions containing 7% w/v and 15% w/v sugar.

5. Prepare an ointment containing 2.5% w/w of API from two ointments containing 1% w/w and 5% w/w of API. 50 g of ointment containing 1% w/w of API is provided.

6. Calculate the amount of ointment containing 5% w/w of API to be mixed with 50 g of another ointment to get the ointment with concentration 2.5% w/w of API.

9 Density, Specific Gravity and Specific Volume

Density is defined as the mass per unit volume of a substance. It is expressed as grams per millimetre or cubic centimetre. It can be determined by dividing mass of a substance by the volume occupied that given mass of the substance.

- *Absolute density:* It is the ratio of the mass of the substance in a vacuum to the volume of the substance for the given mass at a specific temperature.
- *Apparent density:* It is the ratio of the mass of the substance in air to the volume of the substance for the given mass at a specific temperature.
- *Relative density:* It is the ratio of density of a substance at specific temperature to the density of water at 4 °C taken as unity.

Specific gravity is a ratio of the weight of a substance to the weight of water for an equal volume of both the substances at a specific temperature.

Specific volume is a ratio of the volume of a substance to the volume of water for an equal given mass of the both the substances at a specific temperature.

To find out the density of a substance

Q. 1 ml of a liquid weighs 1.1245 g. What is the density of the liquid?

Solution:

$$\text{Density of the liquid} = \frac{1.1245}{1} = 1.1245 \text{ g per ml}$$

To find out the specific gravity of a substance

Q. Find out the specific gravity of a liquid which weighs 24.2816 g for 25 ml.

Solution:

Volume of the liquid = 25 ml

Weight of the liquid = 24.2816 g

25 ml of water weigh 25 g

$$\text{Specific gravity of liquid} = \frac{24.2816}{25} = 0.9712$$

Q. The weight of a pycnometer is 27.8427 g. When filled with a liquid formulation it weighs 57.1291 g. When filled with water, it weighs 52.8409 g at the same temperature. Find out the specific gravity of the liquid formulation.

Solution:

The weight of the liquid = (57.1291 – 27.8427) g = 29.2864 g

The weight of water = (52.8409 – 27.8427) g = 24.9982 g

$$\text{Specific gravity of the liquid formulation} = \frac{29.2864}{24.9982}$$

$$= 1.1715$$

To find out the specific gravity of a substance using principle of Archimedes

Q. A piece of glass weighs 25.4248 g in air. When immersed in water, it weighs 17.2568 g. Find out the specific gravity of the glass?

Solution:

Weight of displaced water = 25.4248 – 17.2568 = 8.168 g

$$\text{Specific gravity of the glass} = \frac{25.4248}{8.168} = 3.1127$$

Q. A glass plummet weighs 11.58 g in air. When immersed in oil and water, weights of the glass plummet are 7.86 g and 7.32 g respectively. Find out the specific gravity of the oil.

Solution:

Weight of the displaced oil = 11.58 – 7.86 = 3.72 g

Weight of displaced water = 11.58 – 7.32 = 4.26 g

$$\text{Specific gravity of the oil} = \frac{3.72}{4.26} = 0.8732$$

To find out the specific gravity of water soluble solid and heavier than water

Q. *A chemical crystal of a salt weighs 4.58 g in air and 2.26 g when immersed in oil. The specific gravity of oil is 0.874. Find out the specific gravity of the chemical salt?*

Solution:

Weight of the displaced oil = 4.58 – 2.26 = 2.32 g

Therefore, 2.32 g of the oil corresponds to 0.874.Let us consider the specific gravity of the salt is X.

$$\frac{X}{0.847} = \frac{4.58}{2.32}$$

$$X = \frac{4.58 \times 0.847}{2.32} = 1.672$$

To find out the specific gravity of water insoluble solid and lighter than water

Q. *A plastic material weighs 5.36 g in air. A sinker weighs 15.56 g when immersed in water. When both the solid attached together and placed in water, weight of the combined solid is 16.12 g. What is the specific gravity of the plastic material?*

Solution:

Combined weight of both in air = 5.36 + 15.56 = 20.92 g

Combined weight of both in water = 13.42 g

Weight of water displaced = 20.92 – 15.12 = 5.8 g

Specific gravity of the plastic material = $\dfrac{5.36}{5.8}$ = 0.9241

To find out the specific gravity of granulated powder insoluble in water and heavier than water

Q. *A pycnometer weighs 30.2672 g. The weight of pycnometer after filling with 15.3856 g granulated material and filled up with water is 59.8472 g. The weight of pycnometer with water is 55.2522 g. Find out the specific gravity of the granulated material.*

Solution:

Weight of the water = 55.2522 – 30.2672 = 24.985 g

Weight of the granulated material and water in pycnometer = 59.8472 – 30.2672 = 29.58 g

Weight of water and granulated material
= 24.958 + 15.3856 = 40.3436 g
Weight of water displaced by granulated material
= 40.3436 − 29.58 = 10.7636 g

Specific gravity of granulated material $= \dfrac{15.3856}{10.7636} = 1.4294$

To find out specific volume

Q. 50 ml of a liquid formulation weigh 57.28 g. Find out the specific volume of the liquid formulation.

Solution:

Volume of 57.28 g of liquid formulation $\cong$ 57.28 ml

Specific volume of liquid formulation $= \dfrac{50}{57.28} = 0.8729$

Conversion of specific gravity to specific volume and vice versa

Q. The specific gravity of a syrup formulation is 1.1562. Find out the specific volume of the formulation.

Solution:

Specific volume $= \dfrac{1}{\text{Specific gravity}}$

Specific volume $= \dfrac{1}{1.1562} = 0.8649$

10 Adjustment of Tonicity— A Practical Way to Adjust Tonicity of Solutions

DEFINITION

Osmosis: When solvent molecules pass through a semipermeable membrane from dilute solution into a more concentrated solution to equalize the concentration of two solutions is known as osmosis.

Osmotic pressure: It is the applied pressure which stops osmosis process.

Isosmotic solution: Two solutions having same osmotic pressure are termed as isosmotic solutions.

Isotonic solution: If a solution having the same osmotic pressure with specific body fluid such as blood, then the solution is termed as isotonic with that specific body fluid.

Paratonic solution: Two solutions whose osmotic pressures are not same (higher or lower) are termed as paratonic solutions with respect to each other.

Hypotonic solution: If a solution having lower osmotic pressure as compared to a body fluid or any other fluid, then the solution is termed as hypotonic solution with respect to that fluid.

Hypertonic solution: If a solution having osmotic pressure greater than that of a body fluid or any other fluid, then the solution is termed as hypertonic solution with respect to that fluid.

Calculation for adjustment of tonicity

Different methods are available to adjust tonicity of a solution. Methods based on freezing point data and sodium chloride equivalent are most frequently utilized. As tonicity of a solution is related to the colligative properties, any of these properties can be used for determination of tonicity.

Method based on freezing point data

It is commonly accepted that freezing point of blood serum and lacrimal fluid is $-0.52\,°C$. If freezing point of any solution is $-0.52\,°C$, then it will be isotonic with blood serum. When one gram molecular weight of a substance having negligible dissociation (i.e. nonelectrolytes) is dissolved in 1000 g of water, the freezing of point of the solution will be $-1.86\,°C$. To produce a solution which will be isotonic with blood serum, we have to adjust the concentration of the solution such that it will give $-0.52\,°C$ freezing point depression.

a. **For single substances in solutions**
  1. Formula for nonelectrolytes to adjust tonicity:

$$\text{g of solute per 1000 g of water} = \frac{0.52 \times MW}{1.86}$$

   MW—Molecular weight

  2. Formula for electrolytes to adjust tonicity:

   g of solute per 1000 g of water

$$= \frac{0.52 \times \text{molecular weight}}{1.86 \times \text{dissociation factor}}$$

Dissociation factor (i): It is the ratio of number of particles formed by electrolyte per undissociated particle in solution.

Dissociation factor for a salt should be determined experimentally. In many cases, dissociation factor for a salt is unavailable. In such cases if number of ions is known, then following value may be used:

Table 10.1	**Variation in dissociation factor with number of ions per undissociated particle**	
Substance	*Particles or ions per undissociated particle*	*Dissociation factor**
Nonelectrolytes and substances with slight dissociation	1	1
Electrolyte	2	1.8
Electrolyte	3	2.6
Electrolyte	4	3.4
Electrolyte	5	4.2

*Dissociation factor: It is calculated based on 80% dissociation of electrolyte. This value may differ based on actual dissociation of electrolyte.

Calculation of dissociation factor

Let, potassium chloride (KCl) has 80% dissociation. We know that it dissociates in water to give two ions.

So, 100 molecules of potassium chloride will produce

1.	Potassium ions	80
2.	Chloride ions	80
3.	Undissociated particles	20
	Total	180

Therefore, dissociation factor of potassium chloride

$$= \frac{180}{100} = 1.8$$

b. For adjustment of tonicity of solution containing active substances using other substance such as sodium chloride

Conc of sodium chloride (% w/v) $= \dfrac{0.52 - x}{0.58}$

x-freezing point of 1% w/v solution of active or inactive substances (only value is considered, sign is not considered)

Freezing point of 1% w/v solution of sodium chloride solution is -0.58. For other tonicity adjusting substances, the formula can be rewritten as:

conc of adjusting substance (% w/v) $= \dfrac{0.52 - x}{y}$

y-freezing point of 1 % w/v solution of tonicity adjusting substance (only value is considered, sign is not considered).

Table 10.2	Freezing point depression data for active and inactive substances	
Name of the substance	*Freezing point of 1 % w/v solution (°C)*
Atropine sulphate	– 0.07
Boric acid	– 0.29
Butacaine sulfate	– 0.12
Chloroamphenicol	– 0.06
Dextrose	– 0.09
Dibucaine hydrochloride	– 0.08
Ephedrine sulfate	– 0.13
Ethylmorphine hydrochloride	– 0.09
Glycerine	– 0.20
Homatropine hydrochloride	– 0.11
Lidocaine hydrochloride	– 0.063
Lincomycin	– 0.09
Morphine sulfate	– 0.08
Naphazoline hydrochloride	– 0.16
Physostigmine salicylate	– 0.09
Pilocarpine nitrate	– 0.14
Sodium chloride	– 0.58

Example:

1. How many milligrams of sodium chloride are required to adjust the tonicity of 1 % w/v solution of atropine sulphate?

Solution: Freezing point of 1 % w/v solution of atropine sulphate is –0.07 °C. We know that

$$\text{Conc. of sodium chloride (\% w/v)} = \frac{0.52 - x}{0.58}$$

$$\text{Conc. of sodium chloride (\% w/v)} = \frac{0.52 - 0.07}{0.58} = \frac{0.45}{0.58}$$

$$= 0.7759$$

Therefore, the above solution requires 0.7759 g of sodium chloride in 100 ml of water or 775.9 mg of sodium chloride in 100 ml of water.

Method based on sodium chloride equivalent

Using sodium chloride equivalent of substances, one can easily adjust the tonicity of a solution containing two or more substances using sodium chloride solution.

Formula for determination of sodium chloride equivalent:

Sodium chloride equivalent of the substance

$$= \frac{\text{mol. wt.of NaCl} \times i \text{ factor of the substance}}{\text{mol. wt. of the substance} \times i \text{ factor of NaCl}}$$

i factor – Dissociation factor

Table 10.3	Dissociation factor and sodium chloride equivalent of few compounds	
Name of the substance	*Dissociation factor*	*Sodium chloride equivalent*
Anatazoline phosphate	1.8	0.16
Atropine sulfate · H_2O	2.6	0.12
Benoxinate hydrochloride	1.8	0.17
Benzalkonium chloride	1.8	0.16
Benzyl alcohol	1.0	0.30
Boric acid	1.0	0.52
Chloroamphenicol	1.0	0.10
Chlorobutanol	1.0	0.24
Chlorotetracycline hydrochloride	1.8	0.11
Cocaine hydrochloride	1.8	0.16
Cyclopentolate hydrochloride	1.8	0.18
Demecarium bromide	2.6	0.12
Dextrose (anhydrous)	1.0	0.18
Dextrose · H_2O	1.0	0.16
Ephedrine hydrochloride	1.8	0.29
Ephedrine sulfate	2.6	0.23
Ephedrine bitartrate	1.8	0.18
Fluorescein sodium	2.6	0.31
Glycerin	1.0	0.34
Homatropine hydrobromide	1.8	0.17
Idoxuridine	1.0	0.09
Lidocaine hydrochloride	1.8	0.22
Mannitol	1.0	0.18
Morphine sulfate · $5H_2O$	2.6	0.11
Oxymetazoline hydrochloride	1.8	0.20

Contd...

Name of the substance	Dissociation factor	Sodium chloride equivalent
Oxytetracycline hydrochloride	1.8	0.12
Phenacaine hydrochloride	1.8	0.20
Phenobarbital hydrochloride	1.8	0.24
Phenylephrine hydrochloride	1.8	0.32
Pilocarpine hydrochloride	1.8	0.24
Pilocarpine nitrate	1.8	0.23
Potassium chloride	1.8	0.76
Procaine hydrochloride	1.8	0.21
Silver nitrate	1.8	0.33
Sodium bicarbonate	1.8	0.65
Timolol maleate	1.8	0.14

Step I: Find out the amount of sodium chloride required alone to produce isotonic solution with the volume given in the prescription. 0.009 g of sodium chloride per ml of solution is required for preparing an isotonic solution containing only sodium chloride. For a given volume, we can obtain the required amount of sodium chloride by multiplying the given volume with 0.009.

Step II: Find out the equivalent amount of sodium chloride for the other ingredients by multiplying the amount of the ingredients given in the prescription with sodium chloride equivalent of the respective ingredients.

Step III: Subtract the amount of sodium chloride (Step II) from the amount of sodium chloride (Step I), which will give the required amount of sodium chloride to produce an isotonic solution with the given prescription.

Step I–Step II = Amount of sodium chloride required to produce isotonic solution with the given prescription.

Step IV: In case of other tonicity adjusting agents, divide the amount of sodium chloride (STEP III) by sodium chloride equivalent of that agent. It will give the required amount of tonicity adjusting agent.

Example:

1. How many milligrams of sodium chloride are required to produce an isotonic solution for the following prescription?

Pilocarpine nitrate   1%

Sodium chloride   q.s.

Volume makes upto 100 ml with purified water.

Step I: Amount of sodium chloride required to produce an isotonic solution for 100 ml solution,

$$= 100 \times 0.009 = 0.9 \text{ g}$$

Step II: From the above table, sodium chloride equivalent of Pilocarpine nitrate is 0.23. Therefore amount of sodium chloride represented by pilocarpine nitrate is

$$= 0.23 \times 1 = 0.23 \text{ g}$$

Step III: Therefore, required amount of sodium chloride to produce an isotonic solution for the above prescription is

$$= \text{Step I} - \text{Step II}$$
$$= 0.9 - 0.23 = 0.67 \text{ g or 670 mg}$$

Step IV: If tonicity adjusting substance is different instead of sodium chloride, first calculate out the required amount of sodium chloride. After that using sodium chloride equivalent of the tonicity adjusting substance convert the amount of sodium chloride into the amount of that specific substance. As example, for the above prescription tonicity adjusting substance is boric acid instead of sodium chloride. We know that sodium chloride equivalent for boric acid is 0.52. Therefore, required amount of boric acid for the above prescription is

$$= \frac{0.67}{0.52} = 1.2884 \text{ g}$$

Method based on using 0.9% w/v solution sodium chloride

At first, we have to find out the amount of the volume of water required to produce isotonic solution with the given amount of drug.

$$\text{ml of water required} = \frac{\text{g of API} \times \text{E value of API}}{0.009}$$

API – Active pharmaceutical ingredient

E value – Sodium chloride equivalent of the active pharmaceutical ingredient

After preparation of the drug solution, we have to add 0.9 % w/v sodium chloride solution to make the volume as per prescription order.

Method based on molecular concentration

A solution containing one gram molecular weight of non-electrolyte in 1000 ml have an osmotic pressure of 22.4 atmosphere. The osmotic pressure of blood plasma and lachrymal secretion is approximately 6.7 atmosphere. Therefore, amount of nonelectrolytes required to produce an isotonic solution is

$$\text{conc. of drug in (g/L)} = \frac{6.7}{22.4} = 0.3\ M$$

M: Molecular weight of drug

For electrolytes,

$$\text{conc. of drug in (g/L)} = \frac{0.3 \times M}{Y}$$

Y: Number of ions produced from one single molecule of the substance

PROBLEMS

1. Find out the amount of anhydrous dextrose required to prepare isotonic solution with blood plasma.
2. Find out the amount of boric acid required to prepare isotonic solution with blood plasma.
3. Find out the amount of sodium chloride required to prepare isotonic solution with blood plasma.
4. Find out the amount of potassium chloride required to prepare isotonic solution with blood plasma.
5. Find out the amount of glycerin required to prepare isotonic solution with blood plasma.

   [For the above questions find out the amount in terms of g of solute per 1000 g of water]
6. Calculate the amount of sodium chloride required to adjust tonicity of 1 % w/v solution of Lincomycin.

7. Calculate the amount of sodium chloride required to adjust the tonicity 60 ml of 1% w/v solution of pilocarpine nitrate.
8. Find out the amount of boric acid required to adjust the tonicity 25 ml of 1% w/v solution of pilocarpine nitrate.
9. Calculate the sodium chloride equivalent of cocaine hydrochloride.
10. Calculate the amount of sodium chloride required to adjust the tonicity of 100 ml of 1.5% w/v cocaine hydrochloride solution. Also calculate the amount of sodium chloride required to adjust the tonicity of 35 ml of 0.8% w/v pilocarpine nitrate solution.
11. Calculate the amount of dextrose required to adjust the tonicity of 50 ml of 1.5% cocaine hydrochloride solution.
12. Calculate the volume of water required to produce isotonic solution with 0.95 g of boric acid. How will you adjust the volume upto 100 ml while maintaining isotonicity of the solution?

11 Hydrophilic–Lipophilic Balance

HLB SYSTEM

HLB means hydrophile–lipophile balance. This system enables us to assign a number to the ingredient or combination of ingredients in a composition we want to emulsify and followed by finding out an emulsifying agent or blend of emulsifiers having this same number. In HLB system, each emulsifying agent is assigned with a numerical value and this value is the HLB value of respective emulsifier. This HLB value of an emulsifier is an expression of the balance of the size and strength hydrophilic and lipophilic groups of the emulsifier. An emulsifier is assigned with low HLB value (<9.0) when it is lipophilic in character and an emulsifier is assigned with high HLB value (>11.0) when it is hydrophilic in character. Within high and low HLB value, emulsifiers are considered as intermediate.

Table 11.1 HLB range and use

HLB range	Use
3.5-6	W/O emulsifier
7-9	Wetting agent
8-18	O/W emulsifier
13-15	Detergent
15-18	Solubilizing agent

In 1949, William C Griffin of Atlas Powder Company introduced HLB system. Griffin devised the formula for calculation of HLB values of nonionic surfactant based on their hydrophilic–lipophilic proportion. The range of the HLB scale is from 0 to 20. When a nonionic emulsifier is 100% hydrophilic, the emulsifier would be assigned an HLB value of 20.

HLB value of an emulsifier can be calculated from theoretical composition of the emulsifier.

$$\text{HLB value} = \frac{M_h}{M_t} \times 100 \times 1/5$$

M_h – Molecular weight of hydrophilic portion the emusifier

M_h – Molecular weight of emusfier

This is known as theoretical composition method. Sometimes theoretical composition method may lead to vast deviation because chemical name of a emulsifier is an approximation of the actual composition. So, it is better to find out the HLB value by using analytical data obtained after analyzing the emulsifier.

HLB value of a polyol fatty acid ester can be determined by using the following formula.

$$\text{HLB} = 20 \times \left(1 - \frac{S}{A}\right)$$

Where S – Saponification value of the ester

A – Acid value of the fatty acid

If the emulsifier contains only ethylene oxide as hydrophilic portion, the formula for HLB determination is given by

$$\text{HLB} = \frac{E}{5}$$

E – Weight percent of ethylene oxide chain

In 1957, JT Davies published an article on emulsifiers and devised new formula for determination of HLB value. He assigned group numbers to various groups of the molecules and calculated HLB value directly from the chemical formula using group numbers.

$$\text{HLB} = \sum \text{(hydrophilic group numbers)}$$
$$- n(\text{group number per } CH_2 \text{ group}) + 7$$

Table 11.2 Chemical groups and assigned group number

Nature of groups	Individual groups	Group number
Hydrophilic groups	$-SO_4^- Na^+$	38.7
	$-COO^- K^+$	21.1
	$-COO^- Na^+$	19.1
	$-COOH$	2.1
	N (tertiary amine)	9.4
	Ester (sorbitan ring)	6.8
	Ester (free)	2.4
	Hydroxyl (free)	1.9
	Hydroxyl (sorbitan rings)	0.5
	$-O-$	1.3
Lipophilic groups	$-CH-$	-0.475
	$-CH_2-$	
	$-CH_3$	
	$=CH-$	
Derived groups	$-(CH_2-CH_2-O)-$	$+0.33$
	$-(CH_2-CH_2-CH_2-O)-$	-0.15

Table 11.3 HLB values for surfactant

Sl. No.	Surfactant	Brand	HLB value
1.	Sorbitan monolaurate	SPAN 20	8.6
2.	Sorbitan monopalmitate	SPAN 40	6.7
3.	Sorbitan monostearate	SPAN 60	4.7
4.	Sorbitan tristearate	SPAN 65	2.1
5.	Sorbitan monooleate	SPAN 80	4.3
6.	Sorbitan trioleate	SPAN 85	1.8
7.	Polyoxyethylene Sorbitan monolaurate	TWEEN 20	16.7
8.	Polyoxyethylene Sorbitan monopalmitate	TWEEN 40	15.6
9.	Polyoxyethylene sorbitan monostearate	TWEEN 60	14.9
10.	Polyoxyethylene sorbitan tristearate	TWEEN 65	10.5
11.	Polyoxyethylene sorbitan monooleate	TWEEN 80	15
12.	Polyoxyethylene sorbitan trioleate	TWEEN 85	11

Table 11.4	Common brand name of sorbitan surfactant
Brand name	*Emulsifier class*
ATMOS, ATMUL, ARLACEL (165 and 186)	Mono and diglycerides
SPAN, ARLACEL	Sorbitan fatty acid esters
TWEEN	Polyoxyethylene sorbitan fatty acid esters
ATLOX	Speciality surfactant: Ionic and non-ionic blend
BRIJ, RENEX (30 AND 36)	Polyoxyethylene alcohols
MYRJ, RENEX 20	Polyoxyethylene acids
ATLAS G-(1086,1702,1726,1441) ARLATONE T	Polyoxyethylene sorbitol esters
ATLAS G-(3300,263,271)	Ionic surfactant

Q. Find out the HLB value of a mixture of 30 g of sorbitan monopalmitate and 70 g of polyoxyethylene sorbitan monolaurate?

Solution:

Percentage content of sorbitan monopalmitate

$$= \frac{30}{30 + 70} \times 100 = 30\% \text{ w/w}$$

Percentage content of polyoxyethylene sorbitan monolaurate

$$= \frac{70}{30 + 70} \times 100 = 70\% \text{ w/w}$$

We know that,

HLB value of sorbitan monopalmitate = 6.7

HLB value of polyoxyethylene sorbitan monolaurate = 16.7

Required HLB value of the mixture

$$= 6.7 \times \frac{30}{100} + 16.7 \times \frac{70}{100} = 2.01 + 11.69 = 13.70$$

Q. Calculate the HLB value of the emulsifier mixture containing 50% w/w of SPAN 20, 25% w/w of TWEEN 85 and 25% w/w TWEEN 60?

Solution:

HLB value of Span 20 = 8.6

HLB value of Tween 85 = 11.0

HLB value of Tween 60 = 14.9

$$\text{Required HLB vaule} = 8.6 \times \frac{50}{100} + 11 \times \frac{25}{100} + 14.9 \times \frac{25}{100}$$
$$= 10.775$$

REQUIRED HLB

Ingredients of an emulsion are assigned with a specific HLB number. This number signifies the required HLB value for proper emulsification of the dispersed phase in the continuous phase. This number is determined experimentally for each oil phase ingredient.

Table 11.5 Required HLB values of some ingredients for both W/O and O/W emulsions

Name of ingredient	Required HLB value	
	For W/O emulsion preparation	For O/W emulsion preparation
Stearic acid	6	15
Lanolin, anhydrous	8	10
Mineral oil	5	12
Beeswax	4	12
Petrolatum	5	12

Table 11.6 Required HLB for O/W emulsions for some emulsion ingredients

Name of ingredient	Required HLB value
Acetophenone	14
Isostearic acid	15-16
Lauric acid	16
Linoleic acid	16
Oleic acid	17
Cetyl alcohol	15–16
Decyl alcohol	15
Lauryl alcohol	14
Oleyl alcohol	13–14
Stearyl alcohol	15–16.
Tridecyl alcohol	14
Arlamol E	7
Benzene	15

Name of ingredient	Required HLB value
Butyl stearate	11
Carnauba wax	15
Castor oil	14
Ceresine wax	8
Chlorinated paraffin	12–14
Cocoa butter	6
Corn oil	10
Cottonseed oil	5–6
Dioctyl phthalate	13
Glycerol monostearate	13
Hydrogenated peanut oil	6–7
Isopropyl myristate	11–12
Isopropyl lanolate	14
Isopropyl palmitate	11–12
Jojoba oil	6–7
Liquid lanolin	9
Lard	5
Lauryl amine	12
Mineral oil (light), napthenic	11–12
Mineral oil, paraffinic (medium), paraffinic	10
Mineral oil (light), paraffinic	10–11
Mineral oil (medium), paraffinic	9
Mink oil	5
Palm oil	10
Paraffin wax	10
Pine oil	16
Polyethylene wax	15
Rapseed oil	6
Soyabean oil	6
Toluene	15

Q. Required HLB value of an oil phase is 12. What amount of TWEEN 80 and SPAN 20 should be mixed to produce 10 g of mixture of required HLB value?

Solution: HLB value of TWEEN 80 = 15(X)

HLB value of SPAN 20 = 8.6(Y)

Let, a and b are the number of parts of TWEEN 80 and SPAN 20 respectively.

$$\frac{a}{b} = \frac{12 - Y}{X - 12}$$

$$\frac{a}{b} = \frac{12 - 8.6}{15 - 12} = \frac{3.4}{3}$$

Amount of TWEEN 80 required $= \dfrac{3.4}{6.4} \times 10 = 5.3125$ g

Amount of Span 20 required $= 10 - 5.3125 = 4.6875$ g

Alligation method is generally applied for solving the above or similar problems.

Q. *Determine the required HLB for the oil phase of the following composition:*

Mineral oil	*35%*
Cetyl alcohol	*4%*
Lanolin, anhydrous	*3%*
Emulsifier	*q.s.*
Water qs. ad	*100%*

Solution:

Required HLB of mineral oil $= \dfrac{35}{42} \times 12 = 10$

Required HLB value of cetyl alcohol $= \dfrac{4}{42} \times 15 = 1.429$

Required HLB value of anhydrous lanolin $= \dfrac{3}{42} \times 10 = 0.714$

Required HLB value of oil phase $= 10 + 1.429 + 0.714 = 12.143$

Q. *The composition of cream requires 4% of an emulsifier blend of TWEEN 80 and SPAN 20. The required HLB value of the oil phase is 13.6. Calculate the amount of each emulsifying agent should be used to prepare 10 kg of cream.*

Solution:

HLB value of TWEEN 80 = 15

HLB value of SPAN 20 = 8.6

Let, a and b are parts of TWEEN 80 and SPAN 20 respectively to get the desired required HLB value.

$$\frac{a}{b} = \frac{13.6 - 8.6}{15 - 13.6} = \frac{5}{1.4}$$

100 g of cream contains 4 g of emulsifier

To prepare 10 kg of cream, amount of emulsifier required

$$= \frac{4 \times 10000}{100} = 400 \text{ g}$$

Required amount of TWEEN 80 $= \dfrac{5}{6.4} \times 400 = 312.5 \text{ g}$

Required amount of SPAN 20 $= 400 - 312.5 = 87.5 \text{ g}$

12

Proof Strength

PROOF STRENGTH DETERMINATION AND ALCOHOL BY VOLUME (ABV)

During 16th century in England, the strength of spirits was determined arbitrarily by observing burning of gunpowder pellet after soaking in spirit. On that basis, strength of spirit was determined. The gunpowder test was replaced by specific-gravity test in 1816; defined as spirit with a gravity of 923 kg/m^3 or $12/13$ th that of distilled water and equivalent to 57.15% ABV at 11°C (51°F), to be as 100 degree proof.

Since, the value 57.15% is very close to the fraction $7/4$ ≈ 0.5714; therefore, for conversion of ABV to degree proof, the value of ABV is multiplied by $7/4$. Therefore, 100% alcohol will be $100 \times (7/4) = 175$ degree proof or 75 degree over proof or 75° OP, and a spirit containing 40% ABV will have $40 \times (7/4) = 70$ degree under proof or 30° UP.

However, the proof system in the United States was not based on specific gravity, instead, it was based on percentage. According to this system, 50% alcohol by volume has been defined as 100 degree proof.

Another proof scale developed by the French scientist, Joseph-Louis Gay-Lussac in 1824, was used in France. Gay-Lussac took 100% ABV to equal 100 degree proof and 100% water by volume to be 0 degree proof. This means that the ABV percentage number is the same as the proof number.

If we compare these three proof scales: Alcohol with 45% ABV is 45 degree proof in France; about 78.9 degree proof in Great Britain; and 90 degree proof in the US.

Another unit is proof gallon. This is commonly used for measurement of amount and strengths of alcoholic solutions.

1 proof gallon =1 wine gallon of an alcohol solution which contains ½ wine gallon of absolute alcohol.

1 wine gallon = 1 gallon by measure

| US gallon | 3.785411784 litres |
| Imperial gallon | 4.54609 litres |

FORMULA RELATED TO PROOF GALLON

1. Proof gallon × 50 = Wine gallons × percentage strength of solution
2. Proof gallon × 100 (proof) = Wine gallons × proof strength of solution

Q. Find out the amount of proof gallons present in 10 wine gallons of 25% (v/v) alcohol.
Solution:

$$\text{Required proof gallon} = \frac{10 \times 25}{50} = 5 \text{ proof gallons}$$

Q. Find out the amount of proof gallons present in 5 wine gallons of 160 proof alcohol.

Solution:

$$\text{Required proof gallon} = \frac{5 \times 160}{100} = 8 \text{ proof gallons}$$

Q. Convert 8 proof gallons into wine gallons of 40% v/v alcohol.
Solution:

$$\text{Required wine gallons} = \frac{8 \times 50}{40} = 10 \text{ wine gallons of}$$
40% v/v alcohol

Q. 16 wine gallon of an alcoholic solution is equivalent to 8 proof gallon of an alcoholic solution. What is the strength of alcoholic solution?

Solution:

Required strength of alcholic solution = $\dfrac{8 \times 50}{16}$ = 25 % v/v

Q. A hospital pharmacy used 30 gallons of 95% v/v alcohol and 10 gallons of absolute alcohol. How many proof gallons were used by the pharmacy?

Solution:

10 gallons of absolute alcohol = 20 gallons of proof gallons

Proof gallon = $\dfrac{30 \times 95}{50}$ = 57

Total proof gallon = 20 + 57 = 77

PROBLEMS

1. Calculate the proof strength of a 75% v/v alcoholic solution.

2. Calculate the percentage strength of 150 proof alcohol.

3. How many gallons of proof spirit are contained in 50 gallons of absolute alcohol?

4. A contain 50 proof gallons of alcoholic solution. If it represents 100 wine gallons, what is percentage strength of alcoholic solution?

5. A manufacturing unit has 10000 gallons of 70% v/v alcohol. How many gallons of proof spirit are represented by the alcoholic solution present in the manufacturing unit?

6. How many proof gallons are represented by 50 gallons 100 proof alcohol?

7. How many litres of absolute alcohol are required to obtain 500 proof gallons?

13

Dry Powder Reconstitution and Units of Protency

DRY POWDER FORMULATION FOR RECONSTITUTION

Dry powder formulations for reconstitution are prepared when drugs are not stable in liquid dosage for a long time. Powders for infusions or injections are sterile and pyrogen free solid substance. When it is to be used, sterile diluent is added to powder to prepare a clear and practically particle free solution or suspension. Penicillin and many other antibiotics are supplied in vial in the form of dry powder. Generally, it is stated in the vial about the volume of diulent to be added to the dry powder. When we are to prepare a solution from the dry powder by adding diluent, we must consider the volume of the dry powder. If it is negligible, we can add volume of diluent equal to the required volume after reconstitution. Such as, a vial contains 10000 units of a drug and desired final concentration is 1000 units/ml. If the volume of the powder is negligible, we can add 10 ml of diulent to produce a concentration 1000 units/ml. Now, consider that the powder content in the vial accounts for 1 ml of the final volume of the preparation. In this case, we have to add 9 ml of water to get a final volume of 10 ml and final concentration of 1000 units/ml.

Q. A vial of penicillin G sodium contains 5000000 units of the drug. If the powder present in the vial accounts for 1.8 ml of final volume, how much of diluent required for preparation of solutions having concentrations 1000000 units/ml, 500000 units/ml and 250000 units/ml?

Solution:

The vial contains 5000000 units.

1. To prepare 1000000 units/ml

   Let 5000000 units of the drug must be dissolved in x ml to prepare the desired concentration.

   $$\frac{x}{1} = \frac{5000000}{1000000}$$

   $$x = 5 \text{ ml}$$

   As powder accounts for 1.8 ml of final volume, therefore, exact amount of diluent to be added = 5 – 1.8 = 3.2 ml

2. To prepare 500000 units/ml

   $$\frac{x}{1} = \frac{5000000}{500000}$$

   $$x = 10 \text{ ml}$$

   Exact amount of diluent to be added = 10 – 1.8 = 8.2 ml

3. To prepare 250000 units/ml

   $$\frac{x}{1} = \frac{5000000}{250000}$$

   $$x = 20 \text{ ml}$$

   Exact amount of diluent to be added = 20 – 1.8 = 18.2 ml

Q. A vial contains 20000000 units of penicillin G potassium. When 75 ml of diluent is added, final concentration of the preparation is 250000 units per ml. What is the volume of powder accounts for final volume of the preparation?

Solution:

250000 units of penicillin G potassium contains in 1 ml of the preparation

20000000 units of penicillin G potassium contains in

$$= \frac{20000000}{250000} = 80 \text{ ml}$$

Therefore, the powder accounts for (80 – 75) ml = 5 ml of final volume of the preparation and final volume of the preparation is 80 ml.

UNITS OF POTENCY

Potency is the measure of drug activity expressed in terms of the amount required to produce an effect of given intensity. Potency of enzymes, vaccines, serums, recombinant, blood products, allergens, endocrines, cytokines, growth factors, toxoid and other biological substances are expressed in terms of units. These substances exist in different forms or preparations. The main objective of measurement of potency in terms of unit is to quantify biological activity of different preparations of the same substance because same quantity of the preparations may not produce the same intensity of biological effect. Generally, each pharmacopoeia defines the units of potency in their own way. WHO expert committee on Biological Standardization expresses potency of biological substances in terms of international unit (IU).

Table 13.1	Few examples of WHO international biological reference preparations
Preparation	*Units of potency*
Activated coagulation factor XI, lyophilized	9.8 IU/ampoule
Amphotericin B, lyophilized	944 IU/mg
Ancrod, lyophilized	54 IU/ampoule
Anti-D immunoglobulin, lyophilized	285 IU (57 µg)/ ampoule
Anti-hepatitis A immunoglobulin, lyophilized	49 IU/ampoule
Anti-hepatitis B immunoglobulin, lyophilized	100 IU/ampoule
Anti-hepatitis B virus "e" antigen (anti-HBe), lyophilized	120 IU/ml
Anti-tetanus immunoglobulin, lyophilized	120 IU/ampoule
Bacitracin, lyophilized	74 IU/mg
Colistin, lyophilized	20500 IU/mg
Dengue virus type 1 RNA, lyophilized	13500 U/ml
Erythromycin, lyophilized	920 IU/mg
Gramicidin, lyophilized	1070 IU/mg
Hepatitis A virus RNA, lyophilized	54000 IU/ml
Hepatitis B surface antigen, lyophilized	50 IU/ml
Insulin, bovine, hydrated crystals	25.7 IU/mg
Insulin, human, hydrated crystals	26 IU/mg
Nystatin, lyophilized	5710 IU/mg

Contd...

Preparation	Units of Potency
Polymyxin B	8403 IU/mg
Recombinant serum transferrin receptor (rsTfR), Lyophilized	21.7 mg/L
Rifamycin SV, lyophilized	887 IU/mg
Spiramycin, lyophilized	3200 IU/mg
Tuberculin, old, liquid	90000 IU/ml
Zika RNA, lyophilized	50000000 IU/ml

SOLVED PROBLEMS

Q. How many millilitres of actrapid (100 IU/ml) are required to obtain 40 units of insulin?

Solution:

1 ml of actrapid contains 100 units of insulin.

100 units of insulin contain in 1 ml of preparation

40 units of insulin contain in = $\dfrac{40 \times 1}{100}$ = 0.4 ml of preparation

Therefore, 0.4 ml of Actrapid preparation should be used to obtain 40 units of insulin.

Q. How many millilitres of human actrapid 40 IU (40 IU/ml) should be used to obtain 25 units of insulin?

Solution:

1 ml of human actrapid 40 IU contains = 40 units of insulin

Let x ml of the above preparation contains = 25 units of insulin

$$\frac{x}{1} = \frac{25}{40}$$
$$x = 0.625 \text{ ml}$$

Therefore, 0.625 ml of human actrapid 40 IU should be used to obtain 25 units of insulin.

Q. A physician prescribes 5 million IU of penicillin G per day for congenital syphilis. Find out how many dose are needed each containing 500 mg provided that 0.6 µg of penicillin G equals 1 IU?

Solution:

Step 1:

$$0.6 \ \mu g = \frac{0.6}{1000} = 0.0006 \text{ mg}$$

$$\frac{x}{0.6} = \frac{5000000}{1}$$

$$x = 5000000 \times 0.0006 = 3000 \text{ mg}$$

5 million IU of penicillin *G* is equivalent to 3000 mg of penicillin.

Step 2:

$$\text{Required doses} = \frac{3000}{500} = 6 \text{ doses}$$

Q. 1 mg of heparin sodium salt is equivalent to 140 USP heparin units. How many micrograms is equivalent to 1 USP heparin unit?

Solution:

1 mg = 1000 µg

140 USP heparin unit is equivalent to 1000 µg of heparin sodium salt

$$1 \text{ USP heparin unit} = \frac{1000}{140} = 7.1429 \ \mu g$$

Q. 1 USP vitamin A unit is equivalent to 0.3 µg of all-trans isomer of retinol. How many milligrams of all-trans isomer of retinol present is equivalent to 50000 USP vitamin A units present in a dose?

Solution:

1 USP vitamin A unit is equivalent to 0.3 µg of all-trans isomer of retinol

$$50000 \text{ USP vitamin A unit} = \frac{0.3 \times 50000}{1} = 15000 \ \mu g = 15 \text{ mg}$$

Q. A patient needs 1.5 million USP units vitamin A units. How many capsules should be supplied to the patient if each capsule contains 15 mg of all-trans isomer of retinol? One unit of vitamin A is equivalent to 0.3 µg of all-trans retinol.

Solution:

Step 1:

0.3 µg of all-trans retinol is equivalent to 1 USP vitamin A unit

$$15 \text{ mg of all-trans retinol} = \frac{15 \times 1}{0.0003} = 50000 \text{ USP vitamin A unit}$$

Step 2:

$$\text{Number of capsules required of vitamin A} = \frac{1500000}{50000} = 30 \text{ capsules}$$

PROBLEMS

1. How many millilitres of actrapid (100 IU/ml) contain 75 units of insulin?

2. A physician prescribes 1 million units of penicillin G daily for 10 days to patient. How much total amount of penicillin is required for if 1 unit of penicillin G is equal to 0.6 µg?

3. A physician prescribes 250 mg of penicillin V four times a day to a patient. Find out how many units of penicillin V is prescribed per day if 1 mg of penicillin V is equal to 1600 units of penicillin V.

4. A physician prescribes 70 units of insulin lispro (100 U/ml) and 32 units of protamine zinc insulin (40 U/ml) to a diabetic patient. Calculate how many millilitres of each formulation should be used to obtain the prescribed units?

5. An ointment contains 5000 IU of polymyxin B per g. Find out the amount of polymyxin B required for preparation of 10 kg ointment if 1 mg of polymyxin B is equal to 8403 IU.

6. A powder formulation contains 250 IU of bacitracin per g of the formulation. How much amount of bacitracin contain in 100 g of the powder formulation if 74 IU of bacitracin is equal to 1 mg of bacitracin.

7. A patient needs to take 100000 IU of vitamin A daily for 3 days. Calculate the amount of retinol should be used to obtain total units of vitamin A for three days?

$$1 \text{ µg retinol} = 3.3 \text{ IU of viatmin A}$$

8. A drug should be prescribed as 15 units/kg of body weight. Calculate the amount of the drug needed by a child patient weighing 60 pounds.

$$1 \text{ µg of drug} = 40 \text{ units of the drug}$$

9. A physician prescribed 250 mg of erythromycin 6 hourly for 7 days to a patient. Calculate the total units of erythromycin supplied to the patient during the treatment period?

14

Calculation of Dose— A Practical Approach for Paediatric and Geriatric Patients

The dose of pharmaceutical formulation varies depending on various factors such as age, weight, disease conditions, etc. Based on these factors, various mathematical formulas (formulae) are used to calculate dose of pediatric and geriatric patients. This chapter includes those formulas to calculate the dose of pharmaceutical formulations. Creatinine clearance is frequently used for dose adjustment in renal impaired patients. Formula related to measurement of creatinine clearance is included in this chapter. Formula for dose adjustment based on elimination half life of drug is also included.

BASED ON AGE OF CHILD

1. *Fried's Rule:* This rule can be applied to infants with age up to 2 years. Age of the patient should be put in the formula in terms of month.

$$\frac{\text{Age (in months)}}{150} \times \text{adult's dose} = \text{Child's dose (approx.)}$$

2. *Young's Rule:* This rule can be applied to children, who are 2 to 12 years old.

$$\frac{\text{Age (in years)}}{\text{Ag (in years)} + 12} \times \text{adult's dose} = \text{Child's dose (approx.)}$$

3. *Cowling's Rule:*

$$\frac{\text{Age at next BD (in years)}}{24} \times \text{adult's dose} = \text{Child's dose}$$

BD – Birth day

4. *Dilling's Rule:*

$$\frac{\text{Age (in years)}}{20} \times \text{adult's dose} = \text{Child's dose (approx.)}$$

BASED ON WEIGHT OF CHILD

Clark's Rule: In this formula, weight of the child patient is considered. The weight should be put in the formula in terms of pound.

$$\frac{\text{Weight of child (lb)}}{150} \times \text{adult's dose} = \text{Child's dose (approx.)}$$

BASED ON BODY SURFACE AREA

$$\frac{\text{Body surface area of child}}{\text{Body surface area of adult}} \times \text{adult's dose}$$
$$= \text{Child's dose (approx.)}$$

The average body surface of an adult person is considered as 1.73 m². So the formula can be written as

$$\frac{\text{Body surface area of child (m}^2)}{1.73 \text{ m}^2} \times \text{adult's dose}$$
$$= \text{Child's dose}$$

Determination of body surface area of a child

(a) *Using the following equation*

$$\text{BSA(m}^2) = \sqrt{\frac{\text{Ht(cm)} \times \text{Wt(kg)}}{3600}}$$

where

BSA (m²) – Body surface area of the patient

Ht (cm) – Height of the patient in centimeter

Wt (kg) – Weight of the patient in kilogram

(b) *Using nomogram:* It is a chart, which correlates the body surface area with height and weight of the patient. Using this chart, approximate body surface area for a patient can be found out.

Calculation of individualized dose of a dosage form

(a) *Based on weight of the patient:* In many cases, dose of a dosage form stated in mg/kg body weight.

$$\text{Dose (mg per kg body wt.)} \times \text{Body weight (kg)} = \text{Dose (approx.)}$$

Body Weight (kg) – Body weight of patient

Dose (approx.) – Dose for the patient

(b) *Based on body surface area of the patient:* If the dose of a dosage form stated as drug/m² body surface area, then dose for particular patient can be calculated as

$$\text{Dose (mg per m}^2\text{ of body surface area)} \times \text{BSA (m}^2) = \text{Dose (Approx.)}$$

BSA (m²) – Body surface area of patient

Dose (Approx.) – Dose for the patient

(c) *Based on weight as well as age of the patient:* The following equation allows to calculate the maintenance dose for any patient (except neonates and infants) to achieve the same average steady state plasma concentration.

$$\frac{(\text{Weight in kg})^{0.7} - (140 - \text{Age in years})}{1660} \times \text{Adult's dose} = \text{Dose (approx.)}$$

Dose (approx) – Dose for the patient

BASED ON TOTAL BODY CLEARANCE

$$C_{ss,AV} = F \times \frac{1}{Cl} \times \frac{x}{\tau} \qquad \ldots(1)$$

$C_{SS,AV}$ – Average steady state plasma concentration of drug

F – Constant

Cl – Total body clearance

X – Dose of drug

τ – Dosing interval

Significant change in total body clearance due to renal disease will effect excretion of drugs through urine. In these cases, desired average steady state plasma concentration of the drug can be maintained in blood by adjusting the dose and dosing interval using Eq. (1).

Determination of creatinine clearance

Creatinine clearance rate determines the normal kidney function. Any significant deviation from normal value indicates impairment of kidney function. So, dose adjustment in renal impairment patient must be done on the basis of creatinine clearance. Different methods are available to determine the creatinine clearance.

1. *Cockcroft-Gault equation:*

   For males,

   $$CrCl = \frac{(140 - \text{patient's age in years}) \times \text{body wt. (in kg)}}{72 \times \text{serum creatinine (mg/dl)}}$$

   For females

   $$CrCl = \frac{0.85 \times (140 - \text{patient's age in years}) \times \text{body wt. (in kg)}}{72 \times \text{serum creatinine (mg/dl)}}$$

2. *Schwartz equation (for neonates and pediatric group to 17 years of age):*

   $$CrCl = \frac{k \times \text{patient's height (cm)}}{\text{Serum creatinine (mg/dl)}}$$

   k = proportionality constant; value for neonates = 0.33 and for adolescent = 0.70.

3. *Sanaka equation (for patients over 60 years of age):*

   For males,

   $$CrCl = \frac{\text{Patient's weight (in kg)} \times [19 \times \text{plasma albumin (g/dl)} + 32]}{100 \times \text{serum creatinine (mg/dl)}}$$

   For females,

   $$CrCl = \frac{\text{Patient's weight (in kg)} \times [13 \times \text{plasma albumin (g/dl)} + 29]}{100 \times \text{serum creatinine (mg/dl)}}$$

4. *By Jelliffe equation:*
For males,

$$CrCl = \frac{98 - 0.8 \times (\text{patient's age in years} - 20)}{\text{Serum creatinine (mg/dl)}}$$

For females,

$$CrCl = \frac{0.9 \times [98 - 0.8 \times (\text{patient's age in years} - 20)]}{\text{Serum creatinine (mg/dl)}}$$

5. *Salazar–Corcoran equation:*

$$CrCl \ (males) = \frac{[137 - \text{age}] \times [(0.285 \times \text{weight}) + (12.1 \times \text{height}^2 \ (\text{in m}))]}{51 \times S_{cr}}$$

For females,

$$CrCl \ (females) = \frac{[146 - \text{age}] \times [(0.287 \times \text{weight}) + (9.74 \times \text{Height}^2 \ (\text{in m}))]}{60 \times S_{cr}}$$

BASED ON RENAL FUNCTION

Renal function is the ratio of the creatinine clearance of patient to the creatinine clearance of a normal person.

Dose adjustment in renal impairment: Pharmacokinetic profile of a drug is altered in a patient with renal impairment. Due to renal impairment, elimination rate and renal clearance are reduced. The elimination half life of the drug increases. This situation poses a problem while selecting a dose for such patients. Based on renal function, dose of a drug can be calculated for these patients.

When the fraction of drug excreted unchanged is below 0.3 and renal function is above 0.7, then dose adjustment is not necessary.

Dose adjustment for drug excreted by only renal route during renal impairment

Normal Dose $\times$ RF = Dose for patient

RF – Renal function

$$\text{Dosing interval for patient} = \frac{\text{Normal interval in hours}}{\text{Renal function}}$$

Dose adjustment for drug excreted both by nonrenal and renal routes during renal impairment

Dose for patient = Normal dose (fraction eliminated by nonrenal routes + RF × fraction eliminated by renal routes)

Dose adjustment based on half life or elimination rate constant

$$C_{SS,\,AV} = \frac{1.44\,F}{V_d} \times t_{1/2} \times \frac{x}{\tau}$$

$C_{SS,\,AV}$ – Average steady state plasma concentration of drug

F – Constant

V_d – Apparent volume of distribution

$t_{1/2}$ – Elimination half life of drug

X – Dose of drug

τ – Dosing interval

PROBLEMS

1. It is given that adult dose of a drug is 150 mg. Calculate the dose for a 10 months old child for the given drug.
2. Adult dose of a drug is 500 mg. Calculate the dose for one year and six months old child.
3. Calculate the dose of a drug for a child 22 kg if the adult dose for the given drug is 250 mg.
4. Calculate the dose of a drug for an 8 years old child if the adult dose of the drug is 50 mg.
5. Body surface area of a child is 0.62 m². It is given that adult dose of the drug is 100 mg. Find out the dose of the given drug for the child.
6. A child born in 26th October, 2003. If the adult dose of the drug is 125 mg, find out the dose of the drug for the child.

7. Dose of a drug is stated as 5 mg/kg. If the weight of a child is 58 lb, find out the dose of the drug for the child.

8. If the dose of a drug is stated as 120 mg/m^2, calculate the approximate adult dose of the drug. Find out the dose of the drug for a 14 months old child.

9. Age and weight of an elderly patient are 70 years and 52 kg respectively. If the adult dose of the drug is 50 mg, find out the dose for the particular patient.

10. Weight and height of a child are 24 kg and 90 cm. Find out the body surface area of the child. If the dose of a drug is 68 mg/m^2, find out the dose of the drug using body surface area method.

11. The weight of a 35 years old male patient is 65 kg. Serum creatinine value for the given patient is found to be 1.9 mg/dl. Find out the creatinine clearance value for the patient. Also find out the renal function for the given patient.

12. Creatinine clearance of a patient is found to be 20 ml/min. The fraction of a drug excreted unchanged in urine 0.65. The normal adult dose of the drug is 100 mg. Calculate the dose of the drug for the above patient.

13. RF value for a patient is found to be 0.42. Normal dosing interval of a drug is 8 h. Find out the dosing interval for the given patient.

15

Basic Biotechnology Calculation

BACTERIAL CELL GROWTH

Bacterial cell growth refers to the increase in number of bacterial cells rather than the size of the bacterial cells. Bacterial cell growth is affected by a number of factors including availability of nutrients, temperature, degree of aeration, genotypes, etc.

Bacterial cell growth has importance in different applications; these are:

1. The yield of a recombinant or cellular protein is highest during a specific time phase of cell growth.
2. Some bacteria are more responsive to bacteriophage infection during a specific period of cell growth.
3. Bacterial cell should be collected at a particular phase of growth for efficient and reproducible transformations by recombinant plasmid.

Procedure for determining cell growth rate

A larger volume of medium is inoculated with a small inoculum of cells. The point of inoculation is considered as zero time. From that point, time is counted for cell growth. The inoculated culture is incubated at proper temperature. At different time points, a small amount of the culture is withdrawn and optical density is measured. Optical density should be measured at 550 nm. A small amount of sample is diluted to give countable number of colonies in solid agar medium in petri dish. If colonies are countable, it can be converted into number of cells in the culture at particular point of time. So, one can correlate the cell number in the culture with time points. It will help to find out the cell growth rate.

SOLVED PROBLEMS

Q. *1 ml of overnight culture of a bacterial strain is inoculated into tryptone broth to make volume 100 ml. 0.1 ml of the sample is diluted with 9.9 ml of tryptone broth. The sample is vortexed, and 0.1 ml of the sample is diluted with 9.9 ml of tryptone broth. Then the sample is vortexed and 0.1 ml is spread onto agar plate. After overnight incubation, number of colonies is counted. The number of colonies is 350.*

1. *Now find out the dilution of cells spread onto the agar medium.*
   Solution:

   $$\text{Dilution of cells} = \frac{0.1}{10} \times \frac{0.1}{10} \times 0.1$$

   $$= \frac{10^{-3}}{10^2} = 1 \times 10^{-5} \text{ ml}$$

   Therefore the dilution of cells onto the agar plate is 1×10^{-5} ml. This means that 10 nl of the initial tryptone broth is placed onto the agar plate.

2. *Find out the number of cells in 100 ml of tryptone broth at the time of sample collection for inoculation onto agar plate.*
   Solution: We know that 10 nl or 1×10^{-5} ml of the sample is actually spread on the agar plate from tryptone broth. Therefore, 1×10^{-5} ml contains 350 cells.

   Concentration of cells in 100 ml of tryptone broth

   $$= \frac{350}{1 \times 10^{-5}} = 3.5 \times 10^7 \text{ cells/ml}$$

   100 ml of tryptone broth contains $= 3.5 \times 10^7 \times 100$

   $$= 3.5 \times 10^9 \text{ cells}$$

3. *What is the concentration of cells in the initial overnight culture?*
   Solution: As 100 ml with tryptone broth contains 3.5×10^9, 1 ml of the overnight culture contains the same number

of cells because 1 ml of overnight sample is diluted 100 ml with tryptone broth. If the volume of overnight culture is different, let 0.2 ml of the overnight culture is diluted to 100 ml with tryptone broth. Now the concentration of cells in the overnight culture is

$$= \frac{3.5 \times 10^9}{0.2} = 1.75 \times 10^{10} \text{ cells/ml}$$

Cell concentration manipulations

Cell concentration can be manipulated using dilution approaches. Mathematical calculations help us to manipulate the cell concentration.

Time after inoculation (h)	Optical density (OD$_{550}$)	Number of cells/ml
0	0.009	1.3×10^7
1	0.024	2.7×10^7
2	0.065	6.2×10^7
3	0.152	1.3×10^8
4	0.228	3.0×10^8
5	0.302	5.2×10^8
6	0.575	1.2×10^9
7	0.920	2.2×10^9
8	1.424	6.4×10^9

1. At time $t = 1$ h, the cell concentration in the culture medium is 2.7×10^7 cells/ml. 2 ml of the culture is withdrawn at that time and centrifuged. The pellet is redispersed in 10 ml of tryptone broth. Find out new cell concentration?
   Solution:

   Number of cells present in X ml of culture medium = Cell concentration × X

   Number of cells present in 2 ml of culture medium
   $$= 2.7 \times 10^7 \times 2 \text{ cells}$$
   $$= 5.4 \times 10^7 \text{ cells}$$

   As 5.4×10^7 cells are resuspended in 10 ml of tryptone broth, new cell concentration

   $$= \frac{\text{Cell number}}{\text{Volume}}$$

$$= \frac{5.4 \times 10^7}{10}$$

$$= 5.4 \times 10^6 \text{ cells/ml}$$

Therefore, new cell concentration is 5.4×10^6 cells/ml.

Calculation of generation time of cells

The generation time is the time required by cells to double the cell number. When we plot a log of cell concentration versus time graph, a line is generated with first part known as exponential region and second part known as stationary region. The slope of the exponential region can be determined using the given formula.

$$\log N = \log N_0 + Kt$$

$$\frac{\log N - \log N_0}{t} = K$$

N – Initial concentration of cells

N_0 – Concentration of cells after time (t)

Q. The initial concentration of cell in cell culture is 1.2 × 10⁷.
After 2 h, the cell concentration is 2.2 × 10⁸ cells/ml in the
exponential region.

　1. Find out the K value,
　2. Generation time for the cells and
　3. What is the cell concentration after 1 h?
Solution:
　1. Given,
　　　$N - 2.2 \times 10^8$ cells/ml
　　　$N_0 - 1.2 \times 10^7$ cells/ml

$$\frac{\log (2.2 \times 10^8) - \log(1.2 \times 10^7)}{120} = K$$

$$K = \frac{8.342 - 7.079}{120} = 0.010525 \text{ min}^{-1}$$

　2. Now generation time for the cells is given by:

$$\log N = \log N_0 + Kt$$

For generation time the value of N and N_0 are 2 and 1 respectively.

$$\log(2) = \log(1) + Kt$$
$$0.301 = 0 + Kt$$

$$t = \frac{0.301}{K}$$

$$t = \frac{0.301}{0.010525} = 28.59 \text{ min}$$

The generation time for the cells is 28.59 minutes.

3. Given, $t = 60$ minutes

$N_0 - 1.2 \times 10^7$ cells/ml

$$\log N - \log N_0 = Kt$$
$$\log N - \log(1.2 \times 10^7) = 0.010525 \times 60$$
$$\log N_0 = 0.6315 + 7.079$$
$$N_0 = \text{antilog } (7.7105)$$
$$= 5.13 \times 10^7 \text{ cells/ml}$$

Therefore, cell concentration after 1 h is 5.13×10^7 cells/ml.

ESTIMATION OF PROTEIN CONCENTRATION

Determination of molecular weight of protein

The molecular weight of protein is determined by using the molecular weight of the individual amino acid.

Formula:

$$MW \text{ (protein)} = \Sigma\{n(aa) \times MW(aa)\} + 18.02$$

where,

MW (protein) – Protein's molecular weight

n(aa) the number of times each amino acid appears in the amino acid sequence,

MW(aa) – The molecular weight of each amino acid appearing in the amino acid sequence.

Name of amino acid	Abbreviation	Molecular weight
Alanine	Ala	71.09
Asparagine	Asn	114.11
Arginine	Arg	156.19
Aspartic acid	Asp	115.09
Cysteine	Cys	103.15
Glutamic acid	Glu	129.12
Glycine	Gly	57.05
Glutamine	Gln	128.14
Histidine	His	137.14
Isoleucine	Ile	113.16

Contd...

Name of amino acid	Abbreviation	Molecular weight
Leucine	Leu	113.16
Lysine	Lys	128.17
Methionine	Met	131.19
Phenylalanine	Phe	147.18
Proline	Pro	97.12
Serine	Ser	87.08
Threonine	Thr	101.11
Tryptophan	Trp	186.21
Tyrosine	Tyr	163.18
Valine	Val	99.14
	Weighted average	119.40

A rough estimate of molecular weight of protein can be obtained by multiplying the number of acid in the protein sequence with the average molecular weight of amino acid.

Protein concentration measurement at 280 nm

An approximate concentration of protein preparation can be determined by measuring the absorbance at 280 nm. In general, one absorbance unit of the protein preparation at 280 nm is equal to 1 mg/ml of protein in the preparation.

Q. A purified protein preparation is diluted 0.1 ml to 10 ml. Absorbance of the diluted preparation is measured using 1 cm path length cuvette at 280 nm. The absorbance of the solution is found to be 0.560. Calculate the protein concentration in the preparation.

Solution:

$$\frac{1 \text{ mg/ml}}{X} = \frac{1.0}{0.560}$$

$$X = 0.560 \text{ mg/ml}$$

Therefore, concentration of the preparation in the diluted preparation is 0.560 mg/ml.

The concentration of the protein in stock preparation is

$$0.1 \times Y = 0.560 \times 10$$

$$Y = 5.6 \text{ mg/ml}$$

Formula for determination of protein concentration using absorption coefficients and extinction coefficients

$$\text{Protein concentration (\%)} = \frac{\text{Absorbance}}{A_{1\,cm}^{1\,\%}}$$

$A_{1\,cm}^{1\,\%}$ – Absorbance coefficient

$$\text{Protein concentration (mg/ml)} = \frac{\text{Absorbance}}{A_{1\,cm}^{1\,\%}} \times 10$$

$$\text{Protein concentration (molarity)} = \frac{\text{Absorbance}}{E_M}$$

E_M – Molar extinction coefficient

Relation of molar extinction coefficient to molecular weight of protein

$$E_M = \frac{A_{1\,cm}^{1\%} \times MW \text{ of protein}}{10}$$

$$A_{1\,cm}^{1\%} = \frac{E_M}{\text{Molecular weight}} \times 10$$

Determination of extinction coefficient of protein

$$A_{205\,nm}^{1\,mg/ml} = 27 + 120\,\frac{A_{280}}{A_{205}} \qquad \ldots(1)$$

Using Eq. (1), one can determine the absorbance coefficient of protein at 205 nm, and then further one can find out unknown concentration of protein. Knowing the unknown concentration of protein, one can find the absorbance coefficient at 280 nm. If the protein contain unusual amount of phenylalanine, the above formula Eq. (1) will not give proper result.

Conversion of protein concentration from mg/ml to molarity

Protein concentration (mg/ml) = Molarity × MW of protein

Protein concentration measurement (Bradford assay)

Bradford assay utilizes a dye reagent to quantify proteins. The dye reagent is Coomassie Brilliant Blue G-250, which is a protein-binding dye. Reaction between dye and protein takes few minutes to complete. The product is stable for approximately an hour.

Q. A researcher prepared serial dilution of bovine serum albumin in the concentration range from 100 μg/ml to 1000 μg/ml. To 0.1 ml of the solution, he added 5 ml of dye reagent. The mixture was vortexed and kept aside for 2 min. The absorbance of the resulting solution was measured at 595 nm. Then he measured the absorbance of unknown sample solution by diluting 40 μl upto 1 ml and same procedure was carried out (0.1 ml of diluted solution with 5 ml of Bradford reagent). The absorbance for unknown solution was 0.65. Find out the concentration of protein in unknown solution.

Concentration of protein(μg/ml)	Absorbance
100	0.09
00	0.18
300	0.29
400	0.40
500	0.51
600	0.62
700	0.73
800	0.84
900	0.95
1000	1.026

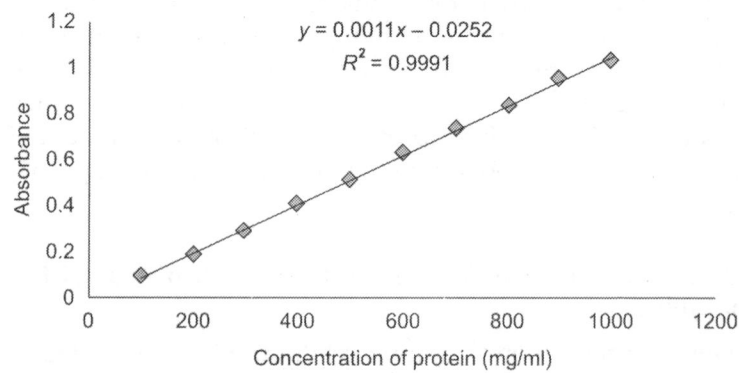

Standard curve

$y = 0.0011x - 0.0252$

$R^2 = 0.9991$

Absorbance for unknown solution is 0.65. Let the concentration of final diluted solution is x.

Now using the equation from the graph, we have

$$y = 0.001x - 0.025$$
$$0.65 = 0.001x - 0.025$$
$$x = 0.675/0.001$$
$$= 675 \, \mu g/ml$$

Concentration of protein in unknown sample using $C_1 V_1 = C_2 V_2$ formula,

$$675 \times 1 = 0.04 \times \text{initial concentration}$$

Initial concentration $= 675/0.04 = 16875 \, \mu g/ml$

$$= 16.875 \, mg/ml$$

NUCLEIC ACID ESTIMATION

Measurement of Double Stranded DNA Concentration

Measurement at 260 nm

Nitrogen bases present in the nucleic acids absorb maximum UV light approximately at 260 nm. Double stranded DNA (dsDNA) shows absorbance approximately 1.0 at 260 nm for a concentration of 50 µg/ml (cuvette length = 1 cm). So, it will have absorption coefficient of 20 for a solution with concentration 1 mg/ml. This relationship is used to calculate the DNA concentration of a sample having unknown DNA content. Quantification of nucleic acid is performed at 260 nm, 280 nm and 320 nm. Absorbance at 260 nm gives specifically nucleic acid content. Any insoluble light scattering components is determine by measuring absorbance at 320 nm. Proteins absorb UV light at approximately 280 nm. The ratio of $A_{260 \, nm}/A_{280 \, nm}$ provides the purity of the purity of the sample. A pure Double stranded DNA sample will have 1.8 as the value for $A_{260 \, nm}/A_{280 \, nm}$. So, the value will be less if there is contamination due to protein. If the value is higher than 1.8, it means presence of RNA in the sample. Pure RNA preparations have a value of 2.0 for the ratio.

Q. Collected DNA from a small culture is suspended in 100 μl of solvent. Then 50 μl of solvent is diluted into a total volume of 2 ml of solvent (Distilled water). The absorbance of the final diluted solution at 260 nm and 280 nm are 0.604 and 0.367 respectively.

a. Find out the initial amount of DNA?

b. Find out the remaining amount of DNA in the initial solution after using 50 μl for spectrophotometry?

c. Find out the purity ratio $A_{260\ nm}/A_{280\ nm}$ for the given sample?

Solution:

a. We know that 50 μg/ml = 1.0 (Approximate absorbance)

$$\frac{C_1}{A_1} = \frac{C_2}{A_2}$$

$$\frac{C1}{0604} = \frac{50}{1}$$

$$C_1 = 30.2\ \mu g/ml$$

Now considering the dilution,

$$V_1 = C_2 \times V_2$$

$$C_2 = \frac{30.2 \times 200}{50} = 1208\ \mu g/ml$$

So, 100 μl of the initial sample contains

$$= \frac{1208\ \mu g}{1000\ \mu l} \times 100\ \mu l = 120.8\ \mu g$$

Therefore, initial amount of DNA = 120.8 μg

b. 50 μl is used out of 100 μl. Therefore, remaining 50 μl contains 60.4 μg of DNA.

c. The purity ratio $A_{260\ nm}/A_{280\ nm}$ for the given sample

$$\frac{0.604}{0.370} = 1.606$$

Using extinction coefficient

A DNA solution has a concentration 1 mg/ml. At neutral pH, the theoretical absorbance for the solution in a path length of

1 cm is 20 at 260 nm wavelength considering G + C DNA content of 50 %. This theoretical absorbance is known as absorption coefficient or extinction coefficient (E).

So mathematically,

$$A_{260} = E_{260}\ lC$$

A_{260} = Absorbance at 260 nm

E_{260} = Extinction coefficient at 260 nm

l = Path length

C = Concentration of DNA solution

Q. A DNA solution has shown absorbance 0.430 at 260 nm. Find out the concentration of DNA in the solution.

Solution: We know that the extinction coefficient is 20.

Therefore,

$$A = EIC$$

$$C = \frac{0.430}{20 \times 1}$$

0.0215 mg/ml or 21.5 µg/ml is the concentration of DNA solution.

Using millimolar concept

The extinction coefficient of 1 mM DNA solution is different from 1 mg/ml DNA solution due to concentration difference. For 1 mM DNA solution, the extinction coefficient is 6.7.

Q. The absorbance of a DNA sample is 0.345 at 260 nm wavelength. Find out the concentration of DNA in millimolarity?

Solution: We know that

$$\frac{C_1}{A_1} = \frac{C_2}{C_2}$$

$$\frac{1}{6.7} = \frac{C_2}{0.345}$$

$$C_2 = 0.0514 \text{ mM.}$$

The concentration of DNA sample solution is 0.0514 mM.

Using PicoGreen reagent

Although measurement at 260 nm for quantification of DNA is a gold standard, it may give erroneous result due to the presence of protein, salt, nucleotides and RNA. So using PicoGreen reagent, one can quantify DNA specifically because PicoGreen specifically reacts with DNA at room temperature on incubation for several minutes. It absorbs light at 480 nm and emits radiation at 520 nm. At first, standard curve must be prepared with known concentrations and then one can find out unknown concentration.

Quantification of single stranded DNA (ssDNA)

In case of single stranded DNA, a solution having concentration (33 µg/ml) will give absorbance 1.0. The average molecular weight for ssDNA is 330 daltons. The optical density (E_{260}) for a 1 mM solution of ssDNA is 8.5 at 260 nm.

Determination of concentration of ssDNA in µg/ml

Q. *A single stranded DNA is isolated from a derivative of a bacteriophage and 20 µl of the preparation is diluted with water to 1000 µl. The absorbance of the diluted sample is found to be 0.670 at 260 nm. Calculate the concentration of the initial preparation in µg/ml.*

Solution: We know that 33 µg/ml gives an absorbance of 1.0.

$$\frac{x}{0.670} = \frac{33}{1.0}$$

$$x = \frac{33 \times 0.670}{1.0} = 22.11 \text{ µg/ml}$$

Concentration in initial preparation can be obtained by using $C_1V_1 = C_2V_2$

$$C_1 \times 20 = 22.11 \times 1000$$

$$C_1 = \frac{22110}{20} = 1105 \text{ mg/ml}$$

The concentration of DNA in stock solution is 1105 µg/ml.

Determination of concentration of ssDNA in pmol/µl

Q. A stock solution of single strand DNA has a concentration of 215 µg/ml. Express the concentration of DNA in pmol/µL. Given the length ssDNA is 6750 nts.

Solution: The calculation process involves introducing conversion factors to get the concentration of ssDNA in desired unit.

$$6750 \text{ nt} \times \frac{330 \text{ g/mol}}{\text{nt}} \times \frac{1 \times 10^6 \text{ µg}}{\text{g}} \times \frac{\text{mol}}{1 \times 10^{12} \text{ pmol}}$$

$$= 2.2275 \text{ µg/pmol}$$

It means that 2.2275 µg of the given DNA is 1 pmol.

2.2275 µg = 1 pmol

215 µg = 2.2275 × 215 = 478.9 pmol

1 ml of the stock solution contain = 478.9 pmol

$$1 \text{ µl of the stock solution contain} = \frac{478.9}{1000} = 0.4789 \text{ pmol}$$

Alternatively we can calculate using a single formula,

$$\frac{215 \text{ µg}}{\text{ml}} \times \frac{1 \text{ pmol}}{2.2257 \text{ µg}} \times \frac{1 \text{ ml}}{1000 \text{ µl}} = 0.4789 \text{ pmol/µl}$$

RNA ESTIMATION

One absorbance unit of RNA is 40 µg/ml.

Q. 10 µl of stock solution of RNA is diluted 1 ml. The sample absorbance of the diluted sample is 0.120. Find out the concentration of RNA in the stock solution in µg/ml.

Solution:

$$1 \text{ absorbance unit} = 40 \text{ µg/ml}$$

$$0.120 \text{ absorbance unit} = \frac{40 \times 0.120}{1} \text{ µg/ml} = 4.8 \text{ µg/ml}$$

Therefore, concentration of RNA in stock solution is

$$x = \frac{4.8 \times 1000}{10} = 480 \text{ µg/ml}$$

Molecular weight, molarity and length of nucleic acid

Molecular weight of ssDNA can be determined using the given formula:

$$\text{MW of ssDNA} = (n_A \times 335.2) + (n_c \times 311.2) + (n_G \times 351.2) + (n_T \times 326.2) + Y$$

where n represents the number of each nucleotide in oligonucleotides and Y value is equal to 40.0 in case of phosphorylated oligonucleotides and -101.0 in case of dephophorylated oligonucleotides.

Q. A ssDNA vector has 5670 bases in length. Calculate 1 pmol is equal to how many micrograms of the DNA vector?
Solution:

The average weight of a DNA base = 330 g/mol

$$\text{MW of the given ssDNA} = \frac{330 \text{ g/mol}}{1 \text{ base}} \times 5670$$

$$= 1.87 \times 10^6 \text{ g/mol}$$

$$1 \text{ mole of ssDNA} = 1.87 \times 10^6 \text{ g}$$

$$1 \text{ pmol of ssDNA} = \frac{1.87 \times 10^6}{10^{12}} \text{ g}$$

$$= \frac{1.87 \times 10^6 \times 10^6}{10^{12}} \text{ µg} = 1.87 \text{ µg}$$

Q. A ssDNA has 4570 base pairs. Find out how many molecules will be represented by 5 µg of ssDNA.
Solution:

The average molecular weight of a base pair = 660 g/mol

$$\text{Molecular weight of ssDNA} = \frac{660 \text{ g/mol}}{\text{bp}} \times 4570 \text{ bp}$$

$$= 3.016 \times 10^6 \text{ g/mol}$$

$$\text{One base pair} = \frac{660}{6.02214179 \times 10^{23}} = 1.1 \times 10^{-21} \text{ g}$$

$$5 \text{ µg of ssDNA} = \frac{5 \times 10^{-6}}{1.1 \times 10^{-21}} \text{ bp} = 4.54 \times 10^{15} \text{ bp}$$

4570 bp = 1 molecule of ssDNA

$$4.54 \times 10^{15} \text{ bp} = \frac{4.54 \times 10^{15}}{4570} = 9.9 \times 10^{11} \text{ molecules}$$

Therefore, 5 µg of ssDNA represent 9.9×10^{11} molecules.
Alternatively,

$$5 \text{ µg} \times \frac{1 \text{ molecule}}{4570 \text{ bp}} \times \frac{1 \text{ bp}}{1.1 \times 10^{-21} \text{g}} \times \frac{1 \text{ g}}{1 \times 10^{-6} \text{ µg}}$$

$$= 9.9 \times 10^{11} \text{ molecules}$$

Q. The molecular weight of DNA is 5.6 × 10⁶ daltons. Find out the number of base pairs in the given DNA.
Solution:

$$660 \text{ daltons} = 1 \text{ base pair}$$

$$5.6 \times 10^6 \text{ daltons} = \frac{5.6 \times 10^6}{660} = 8484 \text{ bp}$$

Q. The concentration of a stock solution of bacteriophage is 4 × 10¹¹ phage/ml. The volume of the stock solution is 10 ml. Now the stock volume is used to purify DNA and percentage recovery of the purified DNA is 90%. How many micrograms of DNA is obtained?

Given (the bacteriophage DNA is 36708 bp in length)
Solution:

$$\text{The total number of phage} = \frac{4 \times 10^{11} \text{ phage}}{\text{ml}} \times 10 \text{ ml}$$

$$= 4 \times 10^{12} \text{ phages}$$

$$4 \times 10^{11} \text{ phages} \times \frac{36708 \text{ bp}}{\text{phage}} \times \frac{1.1 \times 10^{-21} \text{g}}{1 \text{ bp}} \times \frac{1 \times 10^6 \text{ µg}}{\text{g}}$$

$$= 161.5 \text{ µg}$$

As the purity of recovered DNA is 90%, therefore, actual amount of recovered DNA is

$$161.5 \times 0.9 = 145.35 \text{ µg}$$

Therefore, 145.35 µg of DNA is recovered from 10 ml of the stock solution.

16

Formulation of Extemporaneous Preparations— A Practical Guide

LIST OF EXTEMPORANEOUS PREPARATIONS

1. Soluble acetylsalicylic acid tablets IP
2. Compound acetylsalicylic acid tablets IP
3. Aconite liniment IP
4. Aconite tincture IP
5. Adrenaline malate injection IP
6. Adrenaline tartrate injection IP
7. Strong ammonium acetate solution IP
8. Amoxycillin capsules IP
9. Antacid granules BPC
10. Aromatic spirit of ammonia IP
11. Absorbable dusting powder USP
12. Bael liquid extract IP
13. Barium sulphate compound powder IP
14. Belladonna dry extract IP
15. Belladonna tincture IP
16. Belladonna liniment IP
17. Belladonna liquid extract IP
18. Bemegride injection IP
19. Bentonite magma NF
20. Compound benzoin tincture IP
21. Benzyl benzoate application IP
22. Borax glycerin IP

23. Calamine lotion IP
24. Calcium gluconate tablets IP
25. Aqueous calamine cream BP
26. Calamine and coal tar ointment BP
27. Ammoniated camphor liniment IP
28. Camphor liniment IP
29. Camphor water IP
30. Cannabis extract IP
31. Capsicum oleoresin IP
32. Capsicum tincture IP
33. Compound cardamom tincture IP
34. Cassia pulp IP
35. Cephalexin capsules IP
36. Strong cetrimide solution BP
37. Cetrimide cream BP
38. Concentrated compound chirata infusion IP
39. Compound chirata infusion IP
40. Chloramphenicol opthalmic solution BP
41. Chlorohexidine mouth wash BPC
42. Chloroxylenol solution BP
43. Chloroform spirit IP
44. Chloroform water IP
45. Chlorophenothane application IP
46. Chrysarobin ointment IP
47. Cinchona extract IP
48. Compound cinchona tincture IP
49. Coal tar solution IP
50. Coal tar and salicylic acid ointment BP
51. Codeine phosphate syrup IP
52. Compound codeine tablets IP
53. Aqueous cream BP
54. Cresol with soap solution IP
55. Datura tincture IP
56. Digitalis tincture IP
57. Digoxin injection IP
58. Dill water concentrated IP

59. Effervescent granules BPC
60. Seidilitz powder (compound effervescent powder) BPC
61. Emulsifying wax IP
62. Emulsifying ointment IP
63. Hydrous emulsifying ointment IP
64. Ethanolamine oleate injection IP
65. Eye ointments IP
66. Flexible collodion IP
67. Zinc gelatine IP
68. Strong ginger tincture IP
69. Ginger syrup IP
70. Glycero gelatin suppositories IP
71. Dil. HCl acid IP
72. Hyoscyamous liquid extract IP
73. Hyoscyamous tincture IP
74. Indian gum mucilage IP
75. Indomethacin capsule IP
76. Aqueous iodine solution IP
77. Nonstaining iodine ointment with methyl salicylate BPC
78. Strong iodine solution IP
79. Weak iodine solution IP
80. Ipecacuanha liquid extact IP
81. Ipecacuanha tincture IP
82. Ipecacuanha and opium powder IP
83. Kalmegh liquid extract IP
84. Kaolin poultice IP
85. Kurchi liquid extract IP
86. Strong lead subaceteate solution IP
87. Dilute lead subaceteate solution IP
88. Leptazol injection IP
89. Lignocaine and adrenaline injection IP
90. Liquorice compound powder IP
91. Liquorice liquid extract IP
92. Magnesium hydroxide mixture BPC
93. Magnesium sulphate paste BP
94. Compound magnesium trisilicate oral powder BP

95. Mephenesin injection IP
96. Oleated mercury IP
97. Mersalyl and theophyline injection IP
98. Morphine HCl solution IP
99. Morphine and atropine injection IP
100. Compound myrobalan powder IP
101. Small myrobalan ointment IP
102. Small myrobalan and opium ointment IP
103. Nux vomica liquid extract IP
104. Nux vomica tincture IP
105. Opium tincture IP
106. Camphorated opium tincture IP
107. Oral rehydration powder ORS—WHO
108. Orange tincture IP
109. Paediatric paracetamol elixir BPC
110. Paediatric paracetamol syrup BP
111. Liquid paraffin emulsion IP
112. Paraffin ointment IP
113. Penicillin eye ointment IP
114. Liquefied phenol IP
115. Phenol glycerin IP
116. Dilute phosphoric acid IP
117. Compound picrorhiza tincture IP
118. Piperazine citrate elixir IP
119. Potassium chlorate gargle BP
120. Punarnava liquid extract IP
121. Quinine and urethane injection IP
122. Reserpine injection IP
123. Rhubarb compound powder IP
124. Salicylic acid ointment IP
125. Sodium salicylate mixture BP
126. Salicylic acid lotion BP
127. Shark liver oil with malt extract IP
128. Simple elixir IP

129. Simple linctus BPC
130. Simple linctus, padeiatric BPC
131. Simple ointment IP
132. Soap glycerin suppositories USP
133. Soap liniment IP
134. Compound sodium bicarbonate tablets IP
135. Sodium chloride injection IP
136. Compound sodium chloride injection IP
137. Compound sodium chloride solution IP
138. Sodium citrate anticoagulant injection IP
139. Compound sodium lactate injection IP
140. Stibophen injection IP
141. Strychnine HCl solution IP
142. Syrup IP
143. Sulphur ointment IP
144. Dilute H_2SO_4 IP
145. Tannic acid glycerin IP
146. Talc dusting powder BP
147. Terpine hydrate elixir IP
148. Tolu syrup IP
149. Titanum dioxide paste BP
150. Turpentine liniment IP
151. Urginea tincture IP
152. Urginea vineagar IP
153. Urginea syrup IP
154. Ammoniated valerian tincture IP
155. Vasaka liquid extract IP
156. Vasaka syrup IP
157. Wool's alcohol ointment IP
158. Hydrous ointment IP
159. Hydrous wool fat IP
160. Zinc oxide compound paste IP
161. Hydrous zinc oxide ointment IP
162. Zinc oxide ointment IP
163. Zinc ichthammol cream IP

164. Zinc and salicylic acid paste BP
165. Zinc undecylenate ointment IP
166. Whitefield's ointment IP

SOLUBLE ACETYLSALICYLIC ACID TABLETS IP

Synonym: Soluble aspirin tablets.

Each tablet contain:

Ingredients	Official formula
Acetylsalicylic acid	0.3 g
Citric acid	0.03 g
Calcium carbonate	0.1 g
Saccharin sodium	3 mg

Method of preparation: The material after addition of a suitable lubricant, if necessary, is first compressed into large tablets. These are broken up into granules of a suitable size which are passed through a sieve before final compression, the addition of a further small quantity of a lubricant may be necessary.

Category: Analgesic.

Dose: 1 to 3 tablets (acetylsalicylic acid, 0.3 to 0.9 g).

In the treatment of acute rheumatism, 14 to 24 tablets daily, in divided doses.

COMPOUND ACETYLSALICYLIC ACID TABLETS IP

Synonym: APC tablets.

Each tablet contains:

Ingredients	Official formula
Acetylsalicylic acid, in crystals	200 mg
Phenacetin	150 mg
Caffeine	30 mg

Method of preparation: Phenacetin is mixed with the caffeine, if necessary; a suitable inert substance is added to act as diluents, absorbent, adhesive or disintegrating agent and the material in the requisite degree of fineness, is intimately mixed and damped with a suitable moistening agent selected with regard to its effect on the chemical and physical nature of the material. The moistened material is made into granules by passing it through a sieve. The granules are dried in a current of air, at a suitable temperature generally not exceeding 60 °C, and again passed through a sieve.

The addition of a small proportion of a lubricant to the dried granules may be required to prevent from sticking to the punches and dies during compression.

Category: Analgesic.

Dose: 1 to 2 tablets.

ACONITE LINIMENT IP

Ingredients	Official formula
Aconite, in moderately coarse powder	500 g
Camphor	30 g
Alcohol (90 % v/v), sufficient to produce 1000 ml	

Method of preparation: Aconite is exhausted with alcohol (90% v/v) by percolation. The first 750 ml of the percolate is preserved, the remainder is evaporated under reduced pressure to a syrupy consistency, and it is added to the reserved portion. Camphor is dissolved in the mixture; a sufficient quantity of alcohol (90% v/v) is added to produce the required volume. The mixture is kept aside for not less than 24 h, filtered.

Category: Analgesic, cardiac depressant.

ACONITE TINCTURE IP

Aconite tincture contains not less than 0.045% w/v and more than 0.055% w/v of total alkaloid of aconite, of which not less than 30% consists of aconitine.

Ingredients	Official formula
Aconite, in fine powder	100 g
Alcohol	A sufficient quantity

Method of preparation: A tincture is prepared by the percolation process using a mixture of 3 volumes of alcohol and 1 volume of purified water as the menstruum, collecting only 950 ml of the percolate. A portion of the percolate is assayed and the volume of the remaining liquid is adjusted by dilution with the above menstruum, including sufficient hydrochloric acid to produce a pH between 2.8 to 3.2, so that the finished tincture conforms the standard.

Category: Analgesic, cardiac depressant.

Dose: 0.15–0.3 ml.

ADRENALINE MALATE INJECTION IP

Synonym: Adrenaline acid malate injection

Ingredients	Official formula
Adrenaline	0.1 g
Malic acid (L)	0.073 g
Sodium metabisulphite	0.1 g
Sodium chloride	0.8 g
Water for injection, sufficient to produce 100 ml	

Method of preparation: The sodium metabisulphite is dissolved in 10 ml of water for injection, adrenaline and malic acid (L) is added to the solution, stirred gently until a clear solution is formed. Sodium chloride is dissolved in 75 ml of water for injection. The two solutions are mixed and sufficient quantity of water for injection is added to produce the required volume. Sterilization is done by heating in an autoclave.

Category: Sympathomimetic.

Dose: By subcutaneous injection, 0.2 to 0.5 ml.

ADRENALINE TARTRATE INJECTION IP

Synonym: Epinephrine tartrate injection.

Ingredients	Official formula
Adrenaline bitartrate	0.18 g
Sodium metabisulphite	0.1 g
Sodium chloride	0.8 g
Water for injection, sufficient to produce 100 ml	

Method of preparation: Sodium metabisulphite is dissolved in 10 ml of water for injection and adrenaline bitartrate is dissolved in this solution. Sodium chloride is dissolved in 75 ml of water for injection. The two solutions are mixed and sufficient quantity of water for injection is added to produce the required volume. Sterilization is done by heating in an autoclave.

Category: Sympathomimetic.

Dose: By subcutaneous injection, 0.2 to 0.5 ml as a single dose In the treatment of status asthmaticus and other allergic emergencies, by subcutaneous injection, 0.05 ml per minute.

STRONG AMMONIUM ACETATE SOLUTION IP

Synonym: Liquor ammoni acetatis fortis.

Strong ammonium acetate solution contains 57.5% w/v of ammonium acetate; $C_2H_7O_2N$ (limit: 55.0 to 60% w/v).

Ingredients	Official formula
Glacial acetic acid	453 g
Ammonium bicarbonate	470 g
Ammonia solution strong	100 ml or a sufficient quantity
Purified water, sufficient to produce 1000 ml	

Method of preparation: Glacial acetic acid is mixed with about 350 ml of purified water; ammonium bicarbonate is added to the above solution in small quantities at a time until it is all dissolved. Sufficient of the ammonia solution is added until 1 drop of the resulting solution, diluted with 10 drops of water, gives a full blue colour with 1 drop of solution of bromothymol blue and a full yellow colour with one drop of solution of thymol blue, sufficient purified water is added to produce required volume.

Category: Diaphoretic.

Dose: 1–4 ml.

AMOXYCILLIN CAPSULES IP

Amoxycillin capsules contain a quantity of amoxicillin trihydrate equivalent to not less than 92.5% and not more than 110% of the stated amount of amoxicillin.

Method of preparation: Amoxycillin and additives are mixed by trituration. They are reduced to a uniform and fine powder.

The powder is spread on a tile in such a way that the layer of the powder is not greater than about the 1/3 the length of the capsule to be filled. The body of the capsule is then inverted and pressed into the layer of powder until it is filled. The cap is inserted on the body and the capsule is weighed within the permitted limits.

Usual strength: 250 mg, 500 mg.

Use: Antibacterial.

ANTACID GRANULES BPC

Ingredients	Official formula
Dried aluminium hydroxide gel	208 mg
Magnesium trisilicate	52 mg
Alginic acid	481 mg
Sodium alginate	521 mg
Sodium bicarbonate	177 mg
Sucrose and mannitol q.s. to make	5 g

Method of preparation: All the components are mixed and moistened with appropriate solvent (alcohol, hydro-alcoholic solutions) to form a coherent mass. It is passed through appropriate sieve to get desired granules. The granules are dried by air or at drier.

Dose: 5 g by chewing properly after meal at bed time.

AROMATIC SPIRIT OF AMMONIA IP

Synonym: Spirit of sal volatile.

Aromatic spirit of ammonia contains 1.185% w/v of free ammonia (limit: 1.12 to 1.25% w/v) and 3% w/v of ammonium carbonate (limit: 2.76 to 3.24% w/v), calculated as $(NH_4)_2CO_3$.

Ingredients	Official formula
Ammonium bicarbonate	25 g
Ammonia solution strong	70 ml
Lemon oil	5 ml
Nutmeg oil	3 ml
Alcohol (90% v/v)	750 ml
Purified water, sufficient to produce 1000 ml	

Method of preparation: Lemon oil, nutmeg oil and alcohol (90% v/v) is added to 375 ml of purified water in a still; 875 ml is distilled; then distilled and an additional 35 ml is collected separately. The latter is placed together with ammonium bicarbonate and ammonia solution in a bottle of more than 120 ml capacity; the bottle is closed securely and it is warmed gently in a water bath to 60 °C, shaking from time to time until all the salt is dissolved. The resulting solution is filtered, when cold, passed through cotton wool and gradually the filtrate is mixed with the first distilled portion. Sufficient purified water is added to produce the required volume.

Category: Stimulant.

ABSORBABLE DUSTING POWDER USP

Absorbable dusting powder is an absorbable powder prepared by treating maize starch by physical and chemical means so that it does not gelatinize on steam sterilization. It is white, odorless free flowing powder containing up to 2.2% magnesium oxide.

Method of preparation: 100 g of maize starch is treated with 5 g of potassium hydroxide in 20 g of dehydrated alcohol, followed by 5 g of epihydrochlorohydrin in 10 g of dehydrated alcohol. The mixture is warmed to 40 °C and allowed to dry for two hours. The treatment is repeated and after that alkali is washed off with water. The residue is dried at 40 °C. Magnesium hydroxide is added to the residue after drying where magnesium hydroxide content should not be more than 2.2% w/w. The powder is sterilized by dry heating at 150 °C to 160 °C for one hour or autoclaving at 115 °C to 116 °C for 3 minutes.

The pH of 10% w/w suspension of the powder should be 9.5 to 10.8. The loss on drying should not be more than 12.0%.

Use: It is used as lubricant for surgeon's gloves.

BAEL LIQUID EXTRACT IP

Ingredients	Official formula
Bael, epicarp removed and bruised	1000 g
Chloroform water	15000 ml
Alcohol (90% v/v), sufficient to produce 1000 ml	

Method of preparation: Bruised bael is macerated for 24 h in 5000 ml of chloroform water; poured off and the clear liquid is reserved. The maceration is repeated second and third time for 1 h in each case, using 5000 ml of chloroform water for each maceration and the mixed liquid is strained. The mixed liquid is evaporated to 750 ml, cool, add sufficient alcohol (90% v/v) to produce the required volume. The resulting extract is kept aside for 48 h and filtered.

Category: Astringent, digestive.

Dose: 4–8 ml.

BARIUM SULPHATE COMPOUND POWDER IP

Synonyms: Barium meal, shadow meal.

Ingredients	Official formula
Barium sulphate	1000 g
Saccharin sodium	0.25 g
Vanillin	0.10 g

Category: Diagnostic agent (Radio-opaque medium).

Dose: Barium sulphate, oral route, 300 g in suitable suspension.

BELLADONNA DRY EXTRACT IP

Synonym: Belladonna Extract

Belladonna dry extract contains 1.0 % w/w of the alkaloids of Belladonna herb, calculated as hyoscyamine (limit: 0.95 to 1.05).

Ingredients	Official formula
Belladonna herb, in moderately coarse powder	1000 g
Belladona herb, in fine powder, dried at 80 °C	Sufficient quantity
Alcohol (70 % v/v)	Sufficient quantity

Method of preparation: Belladonna herb, in moderately coarse powder, is percolated with alcohol (70% v/v) until 4000 ml of percolate has been obtained. 20 ml of the percolate is evaporated; the residue is dried at 80 °C. Weight of the residue is measured and the proportion of total solids in the percolate is determined.

Category: Parasympatholytic.

Dose: 15–60 mg.

BELLADONNA TINCTURE IP

Belladonna tincture contains 0.03% w/v of the alkaloids of belladonna herb, calculated as hyoscyamine (limit: 0.028 to 0.032% w/v).

Ingredients	Official formula
Belladonna herb, in moderately coarsed powder	100 g
Alcohol (70% v/v)	sufficient quantity

Method of preparation: 900 ml of a tincture is prepared by percolation process. The proportion of alkaloids is determined in this tincture by assay and if necessary, sufficient alcohol (70%) is added to produce a belladonna tincture of the required strength. The resulting tincture is kept aside for not less than 24 h and filtered.

Category: Parasympatholytic.

Dose: 0.6 to 2 ml.

BELLADONNA LINIMENT IP

Belladonna liniment contains 0.375% w/v of the alkaloids of belladonna root, calculated as hyoscyamine (limit: 0.350 to 0.400% w/v).

Ingredients	Official formula
Belladonna Liquid Extract	500 ml
Camphor	50 g
Alcohol (80% v/v)	500 ml

Method of preparation: All the constituents are mixed together.
Category: Parasympatholytic.

BELLADONNA LIQUID EXTRACT IP

Belladonna liquid extract contains 0.75% w/v of the alkaloids of the belladonna root, calculated as hyoscyamine (limit: 0.70 to 0.80% w/v).

Ingredients	Official formula
Adrenaline	0.1 g
Belladonna root, in moderately coarse powder	1000 g
Alcohol (80% v/v)	sufficient quantity

Method of preparation: Belladonna root is percolated with alcohol (80% v/v) until exhausted and the first 400 ml extract is reserved. Alcohol from the remainder of the percolate is recovered and the residue is evaporated to a soft extract under reduced pressure. The extract is dissolved in the reserved liquid. The proportion of alkaloids in the liquid is determined by the assay. To the remainder of the liquid, sufficient alcohol (80% v/v) is added to produce a belladonna liquid extract of the required strength. The resulting extract is kept aside for 12 h and filtered.
Category: Parasympatholytic.

BEMEGRIDE INJECTION IP

Bemegride injection contains 0.5% w/v of bemegride (limit: 0.48 to 0.52% w/v).

Ingredients	Official formula
Bemegride	0.5 g
Sodium chloride	0.9 g
Water for injection, sufficient to produce	100 ml

Method of preparation: The ingredient is dissolved in sufficient Water for injection to produce 100 ml, filtered and immediately sterilized by heating in an autoclave or by filtration.
Category: Respiratory stimulant (specific antidote for barbiturate poisoning).

Dose: In the treatment of barbiturate poisoning, by intravenous injection, 10 ml at intervals of 10 minutes up to a total dose not exceeding 200 ml.

BENTONITE MAGMA NF

Ingredients	Official formula
Bentonite	5 g
Volume of water to make up to 100 ml	

Method of preparation: Bentonite is sprinkled in small portion on 80 g of hot water in small portion at a time without stirring and allowing wetting of the each portion. It is allowed to stand for 24 h with occasional stirring. After that it is stirred to form uniform magma and purified water is added to make up the volume to 100 ml.

Use: It is used as suspending agent for insoluble medicaments. It is pH should be within 9 to 10.

COMPOUND BENZOIN TINCTURE IP

Synonym: Friars' balsam.

Ingredients	Official formula
Benzoin, crushed	100 g
Prepared storax	75 g
Balsam of tolu	25 g
Aloes	20 g
Alcohol (90 % v/v), sufficient to produce 1000 ml	

Method of preparation: Benzoin, prepared storax, balsam of tolu and aloes are macerated with 800 ml of alcohol (90 % v/v) in a closed vessel for not less than two days with occasional shaking. The resulting tincture is filtered and sufficient alcohol is passed through the filter to produce the required volume.

Category: Protective.

BENZYL BENZOATE APPLICATION IP

Benzyl benzoate application contains 25 % w/v of benzyl benzoate (limit: 22.0 to 27.5 % w/v) of $C_{14} H_{12} O_2$.

Ingredients	Official formula
Adrenaline	0.1 g
Benzyl benzoate	250 g
Emulsifying wax	20 g
Purified water, sufficient to produce 1000 ml	

Method of preparation: Emulsifying wax is melted; the benzyl benzoate is added to the melted wax and mixed. The mixture is poured into sufficient warm purified water to produce 1000 ml and stirred vigorously.

Category: Antiparasitic (Scabicide).

BORAX GLYCERIN IP

Borax glycerin contains borax equivalent to 12.0% w/w of $Na_2B_4O_7 \cdot 10H_2O$ (limit: 11.5 to 13.0% w/w).

Ingredients	Official formula
Borax	120 g
Glycerin	880 g

Method of preparation: Borax is powdered, triturated with glycerin, and warmed gently with constant stirring until solution is effected. The solution is filtered, if necessary.

Category: Bacteriostatic.

CALAMINE LOTION IP

Ingredients	Official formula
Calamine	150 g
Zinc oxide	50 g
Bentonite	30 g
Sodium citrate	5 g
Liquified phenol	5 ml
Glycerin	50 ml
Rose water, sufficient to produce 1000 ml	

Method of preparation: Calamine, zinc oxide and bentonite are triturated with a solution of the sodium citrate in about 700 ml of rose water. Liquified phenol and glycerin is added to the above mixture and sufficient rose water is added to produce 1000 ml.

Category: Protective.

Usual strength: 250 mg, 500 mg.

Use: Antibacterial.

CALCIUM GLUCONATE TABLETS IP

Each tablet contains

Ingredients	Official formula
Calcium gluconate	0.5 g
Sucrose	1.0 g
Mentha oil	0.0015 ml

Method of preparation: Calcium gluconate and sucrose are mixed and granulated. Then granules are dried. To the dried granules, mentha oil is added which is previously dissolved in a small volume of alcohol, then mixed and compressed.

Category: Electrolyte replenisher.

Dose: 2 to 5 tablets (calcium gluconate 1 to 4 g).

AQUEOUS CALAMINE CREAM BP

Ingredients	Official formula
Calamine	40 g
Zinc oxide	30 g
Liquid paraffin	200 g
Self emulsifying glyceryl monostearate	50 g
Cetamacrogol emulsifying wax	50 g
Phenoxyethanol	5 g
Purified water, freshly boiled and cooled	625 g

Method of preparation: Self emulsifying glyceryl monostearate and cetamacrogol emulsifying wax are dissolved in liquid paraffin at 60 °C, add with rapid stirring to a solution of phenoxyethanol in 450 g of purified water at the same temperature and zinc oxide are triturated with the remainder of the purified water and incorporated in the cream.

Indication: Sunburn, eczema.

CALAMINE AND COAL TAR OINTMENT BP

Ingredients	Official formula
Calamine, finely sifted	125 g
Zinc oxide	125 g
Strong coal tar solution	25 g
Hydrous wool fat	250 g
White soft paraffin	475 g

Method of preparation: Hydrous wool fat and white soft paraffin are melted together; calamine, zinc oxide and strong coal tar solution are incorporated stirred gently until cold.

Indication: Eczema and psoriasis and other chronic skin diseases.

AMMONIATED CAMPHOR LINIMENT IP

Ammoniated camphor liniment contains 12.5% w/v of $C_{10}H_{16}O$ (limit: 11.5 to 13.0% w/v) and 6.2% w/v of NH_3 (limit: 5.0 to 7.5% w/v).

Ingredients	Official formula
Camphor	125 g
Eucalyptus oil	5 ml
Ammonia solution; strong	250 ml
Alcohol (90% v/v), sufficient to produce 1000 ml	

Method of preparation: Camphor and eucalyptus oil are dissolved in 600 ml of alcohol (90% v/v); ammonia solution (strong) is added gradually with frequent shaking. Finally sufficient alcohol (90% v/v) is added to produce the required volume.

Category: Antipruritic, carminative, counter-irritant.

CAMPHOR LINIMENT IP

Synonym: Camphorated oil.

Camphor liniment contains 20.0% w/w of camphor (limit: 19.0 to 21.0% w/w).

Ingredients	Official formula
Camphor	200 g
Arachis Oil	800 g

Method of preparation: Camphor is dissolved in the arachis oil in a closed vessel.

Category: Antipruritic, carminative, counter-irritant.

CAMPHOR WATER IP

Ingredients	Official formula
Camphor	1 g
Alcohol (90% v/v)	2 ml
Purified Water, sufficient quantity to make up to 1000 ml	

Method of preparation: Camphor is dissolved in alcohol (90% v/v), the solution is added in successive portions to the purified water; shaking well after each addition. Afterwards, shaking is done occasionally until all the camphor is dissolved.

Category: Pharmaceutical aid.

Dose: 15 to 30 ml.

CANNABIS EXTRACT IP

Ingredients	Official formula
Cannabis, in moderately coarse powder	1000 g
Alcohol	a sufficient quantity

Method of preparation: Cannabis is exhausted with alcohol by percolation process. Alcohol is recovered from the percolate by distillation. The residue is evaporated under reduced pressure at a temperature not exceeding 70°C to a pilular consistency and mixed thoroughly.

Category: Sedative.

Dose: 15 to 60 mg.

CAPSICUM OLEORESIN IP

Synonym: Capsicum extract.

Ingredients	Official formula
Capsicum, crushed	1000 g
Acetone	A sufficient quantity
Alcohol (90% v/v)	A sufficient quantity

Method of preparation: Capsicum is exhausted by percolation with acetone. The acetone is evaporated off and the resulting product is extracted with successive quantities of alcohol (90% v/v) until the insoluble residue is free from pungency. Alcoholic solutions are mixed, most of the alcohol is recovered by distillation and the remainder is removed by heating on a water-bath.

Category: Carminative.

Dose: 0.6 to 2 mg.

CAPSICUM TINCTURE IP

Ingredients	Official formula
Capsicum, in moderately coarse powder	50 g
Alcohol (60% v/v)	1000 ml

Method of preparation: Capsicum, in moderately coarse powder is macerated with alcohol (60% v/v).

Category: Carminative.

Dose: 0.3 to 1 ml.

COMPOUND CARDAMOM TINCTURE IP

Ingredients	Official formula
Cardamom seeds, in moderately coarse powder	14 g
Caraway, in moderately coarse powder	14 g
Cinnamon, in moderately coarse powder	28 g
Amaranth	5 g
Glycerin	50 ml
Alcohol (45% v/v), sufficient to produce 1000 ml	

Method of preparation: The mixed powders is moistened with a sufficient volume of alcohol (45% v/v) and 900 ml of tincture is prepared by percolation. Glycerin, amaranth are added to above tincture and sufficient alcohol (45% v/v) is added to produce 1000 ml. Filtration should be done if necessary.

Category: Carminative.

Dose: 2 to 4 ml.

CASSIA PULP IP

Ingredients	Official formula
Cassia fruit	1000 g
Purified water	A sufficient quantity

Method of preparation: Cassia fruit is crushed and the pulp is dissolved out by percolation with purified water. The percolate is strained and evaporated on the water-bath to the consistency of a soft extract.

Category: Laxative.

Dose: 4 to 8 g.

CEPHALEXIN CAPSULES IP

Cephalexin capsules contain the equivalent of not less than 90 % and not more than 120 % of the stated amount of Cephalexin.

Method of preparation: Cephalexin and additives are mixed by trituration. They are reduced to a uniform and fine powder. The powder is spread on a tile in such a way that the layer of the powder is not greater than about the 1/3 the length of the capsule to be filled. The body of the capsule is then inverted and pressed into the layer of powder until it is filled. The cap is inserted on the body and the capsule is weighed within the permitted limits.

Usual strength: 250 mg, 500 mg.

Use: Antibacterial.

STRONG CETRIMIDE SOLUTION BP

It is an alcoholic solution of cetrimide. It contains 20 to 40 % w/v of cetrimide.

Ingredients	Official formula
Cetrimide	20-40 g
Ethanol, sufficient to produce	1000 ml

CETRIMIDE CREAM BP

Ingredients	Official formula
Cetrimide	5 g
Cetostearyl alcohol	50 g
Liquid paraffin	500 g
Purified water, freshly boiled and cooled sufficient to produce 1000 g	

Method of preparation: Cetostearyl alcohol is dissolved in the liquid paraffin with the aid of gentle heat. Cetrimide is dissolved in purified water at the same temperature and added to the warm oily phase. It is stirred gently until cold.

Use: As antiseptic for topical use on skin, ulcers and wounds.

CONCENTRATED COMPOUND CHIRATA INFUSION IP

Ingredients	Official formula
Chirata, cut small	1000 g
Dried orange peel, thinly sliced	100 g
Lemon peel, thinly sliced	200 g
Alcohol (25 % v/v)	1200 ml

Method of preparation: Chirata, dried orange peel and lemon peel are macerated in a covered vessel for 48 h with 800 ml of alcohol (25% v/v). The liquid is pressed out. To the pressed marc, 400 ml of alcohol (25% v/v) is added, macerated for 24 h and pressed. The liquid is added to the product of first pressing. The resulting infusion is kept aside for not less than 14 days and filtered.

Category: Bitter and tonic.

Dose: 2 to 4 ml.

COMPOUND CHIRATA INFUSION IP

Ingredients	Official formula
Concentrated compound chirata infusion	125 ml
Purified water, sufficient to produce 1000 ml	

Category: Bitter and tonic.

Dose: 15 to 30 ml.

For dispensing purposes compound chirata infusion should be used within 12 h of its preparation.

CHLORAMPHENICOL OPHTHALMIC SOLUTION BP

Ingredients	Official formula
Chloroamphenicol	3 g
Kollidon 25	15 g
Preservatives	qs
Purified water sufficient to make up to 100 ml	

Method of preparation: 90 ml of the purified water is heated to 90 °C. After that preservative is added. Subsequently, Kollidon 25 is added and dissolved. Chloroamphenicol is added at last and stirred until it is dissolved. The solution is filtered through 0.22 µm filter paper.

CHLOROHEXIDINE MOUTH WASH BPC

Ingredients	Official formula
Chlorhexidine gluconate	0.2 g
Alcohol (95%)	7 ml
Sufficient purified water to make up the volume up to 100 ml	

Method of preparation: Chlorhexidine gluconate is dissolved in purified water and required amount of alcohol is added. The volume of the solution is made up to 100 ml.

CHLOROXYLENOL SOLUTION BP

Ingredients	Official formula
Chloroxylenol	50 g
Potassium hydroxide	13.6 g
Oleic acid	7.5 g
Castor oil	63 g
Terpineol	100 ml
Ethanol (96%)	200 ml
Purified water, freshly boiled and cooled sufficient to produce 1000 ml	

Method of preparation: Potassium hydroxide is dissolved in 15 ml of purified water, a solution of the castor oil in 63 ml of ethanol (96%) is added, mixed, allowed to stand for 1 h or until a small portion of the mixture remains clear when diluted with 19 times its volume of purified water and then the oleic acid is added. The terpineol is mixed with a solution of the chloroxylenol in the remainder of ethanol (96%), poured into the soap solution and sufficient purified water is added to produce 1000 ml.

Indication: Antiseptic and germicidal.

Dose: 1 teaspoonful solution should be diluted with 250 ml of water and the applied to the affected part for antiseptic protection.

CHLOROFORM SPIRIT IP

Ingredients	Official formula
Chloroform	50 ml
Alcohol (90% v/v), sufficient to produce 1000 ml	

Method of preparation: 50 ml of required chloroform is mixed with sufficient alcohol (90% v/v) to produce 1000 ml.

Category: Pharmaceutical aid.

Dose: 0.3 to 1 ml.

CHLOROFORM WATER IP

Ingredients	Official formula
Chloroform	2.5 ml
Purified water, sufficient to produce 1000 ml	

Method of preparation: Chloroform is dissolved in purified water by shaking.

Category: Pharmaceutical aid.

Dose: 15 to 30 ml.

CHLOROPHENOTHANE APPLICATION IP

Synonyms: DDT application, Dicophane application.

Chlorophenothane application contains 2.17% w/w of $C_{14}H_9Cl_5$ (limit: 1.86 to 2.48% w/w).

Ingredients	Official formula
Chlorophenothane	20 g
Emulsifying wax	40 g
Xylene	150 ml
Citronella oil	5 ml
Purified water, sufficient to produce 1000 ml	

Method of preparation: Chlorophenothane and citronella oil is dissolved in the xylene. The solution is mixed with emulsifying wax, previously melted at a low temperature, poured into the purified water which has previously been warmed to the same temperature and stirred thoroughly.

Category: Anthropod toxicant.

CHRYSAROBIN OINTMENT IP

Ingredients	Official formula
Chrysarobin	60 g
Chloroform	70 g
Simple ointment	270 g

Method of preparation: Chrysarobin is triturated with chloroform; the previously melted simple ointment is gradually incorporated with stirring until the mixture congeals. Loss of chloroform by evaporation is avoided as far as possible.

Category: Parasiticide.

CINCHONA EXTRACT IP

Cinchona extract contains 10 percent of total alkaloids of cinchona (limit: 9.5 to 10.5% w/w).

Ingredients	Official formula
Cinchona, in moderately fine powder	1000 g
Calcium hydroxide	A sufficient quantity
Glycerin	A sufficient quantity
Alcohol (90% v/v)	A sufficient quantity

Method of preparation: Cinchona powder is treated with calcium hydroxide and exhausted with alcohol (90% v/v) by percolation. Alcohol is removed from the percolate; 100 ml of glycerin is added and evaporated to the consistency of a soft extract. The proportion of alkaloids in the extract is determined by assay. Either evaporation of the remainder of the extract or dilution is done to it with sufficient glycerin, to produce an extract of the required strength.

Category: Antimalarial.

Dose: 0.12 to 0.5 g.

COMPOUND CINCHONA TINCTURE IP

Compound cinchona tincture contains 0.5% w/v of total alkaloids of cinchona (limit: 0.475 to 0.525% w/v).

Ingredients	Official formula
Cinchona extract	50 g
Dried orange peel, cut small	50 g
Aristolochia, in moderately fine powder	25 g
Amaranth	2 g
Alcohol (90% v/v), sufficient to produce 1000 ml	

Method of preparation: Dried orange peel, aristolochia and amaranth are mixed with 900 ml of the alcohol (70% v/v) and kept aside in a closed vessel for seven days, shaking occasionally. The above mixture is strained and the marc is pressed. Liquids are mixed and the cinchona extract is dissolved in the mixed liquids. Sufficient alcohol (70% v/v) is added to produce the required volume. The resulting tincture is kept aside for not less than forty-eight hours and filtered.

Category: Anti-malarial.

Dose: 2 to 4 ml.

Compound cinchona tincture contains in 4 ml 0.02 g of the alkaloids of cinchona.

COAL TAR SOLUTION IP

Ingredients	Official formula
Prepare Coal Tar	200 g
Quillaia, in moderately coarse powder	100 g
Alcohol (90% v/v), sufficient to produce 1000 ml	

Method of preparation: Prepared coal tar and quillaia are macerated with 800 ml of alcohol (90% v/v) for seven days in a closed vessel with occasional agitation. The above mixture is filtered; sufficient alcohol (90% v/v) is passed through the filter to produce the required volume.

In making coal tar solution, the alcohol (90% v/v) may be replaced by specifically denatured spirit diluted so as to be of equivalent alcoholic strength.

Category: Disinfectant.

COAL TAR AND SALICYLIC ACID OINTMENT BP

Ingredients	Official formula
Coal tar	20 g
Polysorbate 80	40 g
Salicylic acid	20 g
Emulsifying wax	114 g
White soft paraffin	190 g
Coconut oil	540 g
Liquid paraffin	76 g

Method of preparation: The coal tar is dispersed in the polysorbate 80; salicylic acid is incorporated and mixed with the previously melted emulsifying wax. Separately, the white soft paraffin and coconut oil are melted, the liquid paraffin warmed to the same temperature is incorporated and with stirring, the resulting solution is added to the coal tar dispersion. Mixed and stirred until cold.

Indication: Eczema, psoriasis and other parasitic skin disorders

CODEINE PHOSPHATE SYRUP IP

Synonym: Codeine syrup.

Ingredients	Official formula
Codeine phosphate	5 g
Chloroform spirit	25 ml
Purified water	15 ml
Syrup, sufficient to produce 1000 ml	

Method of preparation: Codeine phosphate is dissolved in purified water, mixed with 750 ml of syrup and the chloroform spirit. Sufficient syrup is added to produce 1000 ml.

Codeine phosphate syrup contains 0.5% w/v of codeine phosphate, $C_{18}H_{21}O_3N$, $H_3PO_4.\frac{1}{2} H_2O$ (limit: 0.48 to 0.52% w/v).

Category: Analgesic, antitussive.

Dose: 1 to 8 ml.

COMPOUND CODEINE TABLETS IP

Ingredients	Official formula
Acetylsalicylic acid	0.25 g
Phenacetin	0.25 g
Codeine phosphate	8 mg

Method of preparation: Acetylsalicylic acid, phenacetin and codeine phosphate are mixed. The material after addition of a suitable lubricant, if necessary, is first compressed into large tablets. These are broken up into granules of a suitable size which are passed through a sieve before final compression, the addition of a further small quantity of a lubricant may be necessary.

Category: Antipyretic, analgesic.

Dose: 1 or 2 tablets.

AQUEOUS CREAM BP

Ingredients	Official formula
Emulsifying ointment	300 g
Phenoxyethanol	10 g
Purified water, freshly boiled and cooled	690 g

Method of preparation: Phenoxyethanol is dissolved in the purified water with gentle heating. Phenoxyethanol solution is added to melted emulsifying ointment while warm. The mixture stirred is until cold.

Use: Pharmaceutical aid.

CRESOL WITH SOAP SOLUTION IP

Synonym: Lysol

Cresol with soap solution contains 50% v/v of cresol (limit: 47.0 to 53.0% v/v). It is prepared by the saponification of a mixture of cresol with vegetable oils or the mixed fatty acids derived there from, excluding coconut and palm kernel oils. The vegetable oil may be cottonseed, linseed or soyabean or similar oils, which have a saponification value not greater than 205 and an iodine value not less than 100.

Ingredients	Official formula
Cresol	500 ml
Vegetable oil	180 g
Potassium hydroxide	42 g
Purified water, sufficient to produce 1000 ml	

Method of preparation: Potassium hydroxide is dissolved in 250 ml of purified water; the vegetable oil is added and heated on a water-bath. Mixing is done thoroughly and heating is continued until a small portion dissolves in water without the separation of oily drops. Cresol is added and mixed thoroughly. Sufficient purified water is added to produce the required volume.

Category: Disinfectant.

DATURA TINCTURE IP

Datura tincture contains 0.025% w/v of the alkaloids of datura herb, calculated as hyoscyamine (limit: 0.0225 to 0.0275% w/v).

Ingredients	Official formula
Datura liquid extract	100 ml
Alcohol (45% v/v) sufficient to produce 1000 ml	

Method of preparation: Datura liquid extract and alcohol (45% v/v) are mixed. The above mixture is kept aside for not less than twelve hours and filtered.

Category: Parasympatholytic.

Dose: 0.3 to 2 ml.

In the treatment of parkinsonism, dose is 2 to 16 ml.

Datura tincture contains in 2 ml 0.5 mg of the alkaloids of datura herb, calculated as hyoscyamine.

DIGITALIS TINCTURE IP

1. *Preparation from digitalis:*

Ingredients	Official formula
Digitalis, in moderately coarse powder	100 g
Alcohol (70% v/v)	A sufficient quantity

Method of preparation: 700 ml of a tincture is prepared by the percolation process. To the remainder portion of the tincture, sufficient quantity of Alcohol (70% v/v) is added to produce a digitalis tincture of required strength.

2. *Preparation from prepared digitalis:*

Ingredients	Official formula
Prepared digitalis	A quantity containing 1000 unit of activity
Alcohol (70% v/v) sufficient to produce 1000 ml	

Method of preparation: Prepared digitalis is macerated with alcohol (70% v/v) in a close vessel for two days, shaking occasionally. After maceration, straining is done and the marc is pressed lightly. Mixing of the liquids is done followed by filtration. Volume of the tincture is adjusted with alcohol (70% v/v).

Category: Cardiotonic.

Dose: 0.3 to 1 ml.

DIGOXIN INJECTION IP

Digoxin injection contains not less than 0.0225% w/v and not more than 0.0275% w/v of digoxin.

Ingredients	Official formula
Digoxin	25 mg
Alcohol (80% v/v)	12.5 ml
Propylene glycol	40 ml
Citric acid	75 mg
Sodium phosphate	0.45 mg
Water for injection, sufficient to produce 100 ml	

Method of preparation: Digoxin is dissolved in the alcohol (80% v/v). To the above solution, propylene glycol, a solution of the citric acid and sodium phosphate in water for injection is added. Sufficient water for injection is added to produce 100 ml. The above injection is distributed in ampoules and sterilized by heating in an autoclave.

Category: Cardiotonic

Dose: By intramuscular or slow intravenous injection 2 to 4 ml. Digoxin injection contains 1 mg of digoxin in 4 ml.

DILL WATER CONCENTRATED IP

Ingredients	Official formula
Dill oil	20 ml
Alcohol (90% v/v)	600 ml
Purified water, sufficient to produce 1000 ml	

Method of preparation: Dill oil is dissolved in alcohol (90% v/v). Sufficient purified water is added in successive small quantities with vigorous shaking after each addition to produce 1000 ml. 50 g of talc powder is added to the above solution and it is mixed by shaking. The mixture is kept aside for a few hours, shaking occasionally and filtered.

Category: Carminative, flavoring agent.

Dose: 0.3 to 1 ml.

EFFERVESCENT GRANULES BPC

Ingredients	Official formula
Sodium bicarbonate	55.3 g
Citric acid	31.3 g
Tartaric acid	3.6 g

Ingredients	Official formula
Calcium lactate	3.6 g
Potassium bicarbonate	3.6 g
Sodium chloride	1.8 g
Sodium phosphate	0.4 g

Method of preparation: All the components are mixed and moistened with appropriate solvent (alcohol, hydro-alcoholic solutions) to form a coherent mass. It is passed through appropriate sieve to get desired granules. The granules are dried by air or at drier.

Dose: 1 to 2 teaspoonfuls in a glass of water trice daily

Indication: Indigestion, flatulence, hyperacidity, gastric irritation, acidosis, nephritis, headache, toxaemia of pregnancy.

SEIDILITZ POWDER BPC (COMPOUND EFFERVESCENT POWDER)

It consists of two different powders.

Powder A

Ingredients	Official formula
Sodium potassium tartrate	7.5 g
Sodium bicarbonate	2.5 g

A fine powder of both the ingredients are made and mixed by the method of trituration in a motar and pestle. This powder mixture is dispensed in blue paper, which indicates that the contents are alkaline.

Powder B

Ingredients	Official formula
Tartaric acid	2.5 g

A fine powder is made and dispensed in white paper.

Mode of administration: The content of the blue paper is first dissolved in tumblerful cold or warm water and then the powder in whitepaper is added. The liquid is taken immediately after mixing.

Dose: 8–18 g

Preferably take in morning hours. It should be used cautiously in patients with cardiac failure, renal impaired patients, toxaemia of pregnancy.

EMULSIFYING WAX IP

Emulsifying wax contains cetostearyl alcohol and sodium lauryl sulphate or similar sodium salt of sulphated higher primary aliphatic alcohols.

A suitable preparation can be prepared by the following process:

Ingredients	Official formula
Cetostearyl Alcohol	900 g
Sodium Lauryl Sulphate	100 g
Purified water	40 ml

Method of preparation: Cetostearyl alcohol is melted and heated to about 95 °C. Sodium lauryl sulphate is added and mixed; purified water is added and heated to 115 °C. Heating is continued at 115 °C, stirring vigorously until frothing ceases and the product is translucent. The product is cooled quickly.

Category: Pharmaceutical aid.

EMULSIFYING OINTMENT IP

Ingredients	Official formula
Emulsifying wax	300 g
White soft paraffin	500 g
Liquid paraffin	200 g

Method of preparation: All the constituents are melted together, stirred until it attains room temperature.

Category: Pharmaceutical aid.

Emulsifying ointment is used as an ingredient of hydrous emulsifying ointment, zinc undecylenate ointment.

HYDROUS EMULSIFYING OINTMENT IP

Ingredients	Official formula
Emulsifying ointment	300 g
Chlorocresol	1 g
Purified water	699 g

Method of preparation: Chlorocresol is dissolved in purified water with the aid of gentle heat. Emulsifying ointment is melted; the solution of chlorocresol is added while warm. The ointment is stirred gently until it attains room temperature.
Category: Pharmaceutical aid.

ETHANOLAMINE OLEATE INJECTION IP

Ethanolamine oleate injection contains ethanolamine oleate equivalent to not less than 3.9% w/v and not more than 4.3% w/v of oleic acid, $C_{17}H_{33}CO_2H_2$ and not less than 0.85% w/v and not more than 0.93% w/v of ethanolamine, C_2H_7ON.

Ingredients	Official formula
Ethanolamine	0.91 g
Oleic acid	4.23 g
Benzyl alcohol	2 ml
Water for injection, sufficient to produce 100 ml	

Method of preparation: Oleic acid is added to 50 ml of water for injection in a closed container with shaking. Ethanolamine is added gradually, shaking between each addition until combination is complete. Benzyl alcohol is added followed by shaking. Sufficient water for injection is added to produce 100 ml. The final product is sterilized by heating in an autoclave.
Category: Sclerosing agent, pharmaceutical aid.
Dose: By intravenous injection, 2 to 5 ml.

EYE OINTMENTS IP

Eye ointments can be prepared with the following basis:

Ingredients	Official formula
Liquid paraffin	10 g
Wool fat	10 g
White soft paraffin	80 g

Method of preparation: Wool fat and the white soft paraffin are melted together. Liquid paraffin is added and the hot mixture is filtered through coarse filter paper placed in a heated funnel. Then the ointment is sterilized by heating at 150 °C for sufficient time to ensure that the whole product is maintained at this temperature for one hour, allowed to cool.

Preparation:

Process 1: Very finely powdered drug is triturated with a small portion of melted basis until the mixture is smooth, sufficient of the melted base is added gradually to produce the required weight and trituration is continued until the eye ointment attains room temperature.

Process 2: Active ingredients are dissolved in the smallest quantity of water for injection and incorporated with the basis as in Process 1.

FLEXIBLE COLLODION IP

Synonym: Collodion

Ingredients	Official formula
Pyroxylin	16 g
Colophony	30 g
Castor oil	20 g
Alcohol (90 % v/v)	240 ml
Solvent ether sufficient to produce 1000 ml	

Method of preparation: Pyroxylin is immersed in the alcohol (90 % v/v), followed by addition of colophony and castor oil. Finally sufficient solvent ether is added to produce the required volume. The product is occasionally shaken until dissolve. The product is kept aside for any deposit to settle, the clear liquid is decanted.

Category: Pharmaceutical aid.

ZINC GELATIN IP

Synonym: Unna's paste.

Zinc gelatin contains 15.0 % w/w of zinc oxide (limit: 14.0 to 16.0 % w/w).

Ingredients	Official formula
Zinc oxide, finely sifted	150 g
Gelatin, cut small	150 g
Glycerin	350 g
Purified wateror sufficient quantity	350 ml

Method of preparation: Gelatin is softened thoroughly in the purified water; glycerin is added and heated on a water-bath until the gelatin is dissolved. The weight of the product is adjusted to 850 g by the addition of a further quantity of purified water. Zinc oxide is incorporated and stirred until about set.

Category: Protective

STRONG GINGER TINCTURE IP

Synonym: Essence of ginger.

Ingredients	Official formula
Ginger, in moderately coarse powder	500 g
Alcohol (90% v/v), sufficient to produce 1000 ml	

Method of preparation: The above tincture is prepared by percolation process.

Category: Carminative

Dose: 0.3 to 0.6 ml

GINGER SYRUP IP

Ingredients	Official formula
Strong ginger tincture	50 ml
Syrup, sufficient to produce 1000 ml	

Method of preparation: Strong ginger tincture and syrup are mixed together, volume made up to 1000 ml with syrup.

Category: Carminative

Dose: 2 to 4 ml

GLYCERO GELATIN SUPPOSITORIES IP

Ingredients	Official formula
Gelatin, cut small	14 g
Glycerin	70 g
Purified Water	A sufficient quantity

Method of preparation: Gelatin is added to 30 ml of hot water (heated nearly to boiling) and glycerol is added. The mixture is heated on water bath for 15 minutes or until a clear solution is produced. The weight of the water is adjusted to 100 g by adding hot purified water or by evaporation of water on water bath as appropriate. The solution is poured into moulds. In case of tropical and sub tropical countries, gelatin requirement may be up to 18% w/w.

Category: Rectal evacuant.

DILUTE HYDROCHLORIC ACID IP

Dilute hydrochloric acid contains 10% w/w of HCl (limit: 9.5 to 10.5% w/w)

Ingredients	Official formula
Hydrochloric acid	274 g
Purified water	726 g

Method of preparation: Hydrochloric acid is added to purified water and volume is made up to 1000 g with purified water.

Category: Acidifier.

Dose: 0.6 to 8 ml.

HYOSCYAMUS LIQUID EXTRACT IP

Hyoscyamus liquid extract contains 0.05% w/v of the alkaloids of hyoscyamus, calculated as hyoscyamine (limit: 0.045 to 0.055% w/v).

Ingredients	Official formula
Hyoscyamus, in moderately coarse powder	1000 g
Alcohol (70% v/v)	a sufficient quantity

Method of preparation: Hyoscyamus is percolated with alcohol (70% v/v) until exhausted and first 850 ml of the percolate is reserved. Alcohol is recovered from the remainder of the percolate by evaporation under reduced pressure at a temperature not exceeding 60 °C; the residue is evaporated to a soft extract at a temperature not exceeding 60 °C and this extract is dissolved in the reserve portion. The proportion of alkaloids is determined in the liquid. To the remainder of the liquid, sufficient alcohol (70% v/v) is added to produce hyoscyamus liquid extract of the required strength. The resulting extract is kept aside not less than 24 h and filtered, if necessary.

Category: Parasympatholytic

Dose: 0.2 to 0.4 ml.

HYOSCYAMUS TINCTURE IP

Hyoscyamus tincture contains 0.005% w/v of the alkaloids of hyoscyamus, calculated as hyoscyamine (limit: 0.0045 to 0.0055% w/v).

Ingredients	Official formula
Hyoscyamus Liquids Extract	100 ml
Alcohol (70% v/v), sufficient to produce 1000 ml	

Method of preparation: Hyoscyamus liquids extract and alcohol (70% v/v) are mixed together. The product is kept aside for not less than twelve hours and filtered.

Category: Parasympatholytic

Dose: 2 to 4 ml.

Hyoscyamus tincture contains in 4 ml 0.2 mg of the alkaloids of hyoscyamus, calculated as hyoscyamine.

INDIAN GUM MUCILAGE IP

Ingredients	Official formula
Indian gum powder	400 g
Chloroform water	600 ml

Method of preparation: Indian gum is rapidly rinsed with a little purified water. Then it is dissolved in the chloroform water in a closed vessel and strained.

Note: Indian gum mucilage should be freshly prepared.

Category: Pharmaceutical aid.

INDOMETHACIN CAPSULE IP

Indomethacin capsules contain not less than 90% and not more than 110% of the stated amount of indomethacin.

Method of preparation: Indomethacin and additives are mixed by trituration. They are reduced to a uniform and fine powder. The powder is spread on a tile in such a way that the layer of the powder is not greater than about the 1/3rd the length of the capsule to be filled. The body of the capsule is then inverted and pressed into the layer of powder until it is filled. The cap is inserted on the body and the capsule is weighed within the permitted limits.

Use: Anti-inflammatory and analgesic

AQUEOUS IODINE SOLUTION IP

Synonym: Lugol's solution

Aqueous solution of iodine contains 5% w/v of iodine, I_2 (limit: 4.9 to 5.1% w/v) and 10% w/v of potassium iodide, KI (limit: 9.8 to 10.2% w/v).

Ingredients	Official formula
Iodine	50 g
Potassium iodide	100 g
Purified water, sufficient to produce 1000 ml	

Method of preparation: Potassium iodide and iodine are dissolved together in the 100 ml of purified water. Sufficient purified water is added to produce the required volume.

Category: Local anti-infective, source of iodine

Dose: 0.3 to 1 ml

NONSTAINING IODINE OINTMENT WITH METHYL SALICYLATE BPC

This ointment contains 4.3 to 5.0 percent iodine and 5.6 to 6.2% w/w methyl salicylate.

Ingredients	Official formula
Iodine	4.16 g
Oleic acid	2.30 g
Linseed oil	1.38 g
Yellow soft paraffin sufficient to produce 100 g	

Method of preparation: Oleic acid, linseed oil and yellow soft paraffin are taken in a wide mouthed bottle. Then finely powdered iodine is added to the bottle. The bottle is stoppered and heated on a water bath (temperature not exceeding 60 °C) with occasional stirring until a dark greenish-black product is formed. The greenish black colour indicates formation of the product. It may take 2 to 6 h for combination of iodine. The whole content is allowed to cool without stirring an opaque nonstaining iodine ointment is formed.

Ingredients	Official formula
Methyl salicylate	50 ml
Nonstaining iodine ointment to make the weight 1000 g	

Method of preparation: The nonstaining iodine is melted at a low temperature and methyl salicylate is added and stirred until cold.

STRONG IODINE SOLUTION IP

Strong iodine solution contains 10% w/v of iodine, I (limit: 9.5 to 10.5% w/v) and 6% w/v of potassium iodide, KI (limit: 5.7 to 6.3% w/v).

Ingredients	Official formula
Iodine	100 g
Potassium Iodide	60 g
Purified water	100 ml
Alcohol (90% v/v), sufficient to produce 1000 ml	

Method of preparation: Potassium iodide and iodine are dissolved in the purified water and sufficient alcohol (90% v/v) is added to produce 1000 ml.

Category: Antiseptic

In making strong iodine solution, potassium iodide may be replaced by sodium iodide.

WEAK IODINE SOLUTION IP

Synonym: Iodine tincture

Weak iodine solution contains 2% w/v of iodine, 1 (limit: 1.96 to 2.05% w/v) and 2.5% w/v of potassium iodide, KI (limit: 2.45 to 2.55% w/v).

Ingredients	Official formula
Iodine	20 g
Potassium iodide	25 g
Alcohol (50% v/v), sufficient to produce 1000 ml	

Method of preparation: Potassium iodide and iodine are dissolved in alcohol (50% v/v) to produce the required volume.

Category: Antiseptic

Dose: 0.3 to 2 ml.

Weak Iodine solution contains in 2 ml, 40 mg of iodine and about 78 mg of total iodine, free and combined.

Potassium iodide may be replaced by sodium iodine in making weak iodide solution.

IPECACUANHA LIQUID EXTRACT IP

Ipecacuanha liquid extract contains 2.0% w/v of the total alkaloids of ipecacuanha, calculated as emetine (limit: 1.9 to 2.1% w/v).

Ingredients	Official formula
Ipecacuanha, in fine powder	1000 g
Alcohol (80% v/v)	a sufficient quantity

Method of preparation: 750 ml extract is collected by percolating ipecacuanha with alcohol with (80% v/v) and this portion is reserved. Percolation is continued till ipecacuanha is exhausted. Alcohol is recovered from this percolate by distillation under reduced pressure at a temperature not exceeding 60 °C and the residual extract is dissolved in the reduced portion. To the remainder of the liquid, sufficient Alcohol (80 % v/v) is added to produce an ipecacuanha liquid extract of required strength. The resulting product is kept aside for not less than 24 h and filtered.

Category: Expectorant and emetic.

Dose: 0.03 to 0.12 ml, *Dose:* Emetic 0.6 to 2 ml.

Ipecacuanha liquid extract contains in 0.12 ml, 2.4 mg of the total alkaloids of ipecacuanha, calculated as emetine.

IPECACUANHA TINCTURE IP

Ipecacuanha tincture contains 0.2% w/v of the total alkaloids of Ipecacuanha, calculated as emetine.

Ingredients	Official formula
Ipecacuanha liquid extract	100 ml
Dilute acetic acid	16.5 ml
Alcohol (90% v/v)	210 ml
Glycerin	200 ml
Purified water, sufficient to produce 1000 ml	

Method of preparation: Dilute acetic acid and alcohol (90% v/v) are mixed with a mixture of glycerin and 500 ml of purified water, ipecacuanha liquid extract is added to the above and sufficient purified water is added to produce 1000 ml. The resulting tincture is kept aside for 24 h and filtered.

Category: Expectorant and emetic

Dose: 0.3 to 1.2 ml, *Dose:* Emetic 6 to 20 ml.

Ipecacuanha tincture contains in 1.2 ml, 2.4 mg of total alkaloids of ipecacuanha, calculated as emetine.

IPECACUANHA AND OPIUM POWDER IP

Synonym: Dover's powder

Ipecacuanha and opium powder contains 10% w/w of powdered opium, equivalent to 1% w/w of anhydrous morphine, $C_{17}H_{19}O_3N$ (limit: 0.95 to 1.05% w/w).

Ingredients	Official formula
Prepared ipecacuanha	100 g
Powdered opium	100 g
Lactose, finely powdered	800 g

Method of preparation: All the constituents are mixed together.

Category: Antipyretic

Dose: 0.3 to 0.6 g

Ipecacuanha and opium powder contains in 0.6 g, 6 mg of anhydrous morphine.

KALMEGH LIQUID EXTRACT IP

Kalmegh liquid extract contains 0.5% w/v of andrographolide (limit: 0.45 to 0.55% w/v).

Ingredients	Official formula
Kalmegh	500 g
Fennel oil	2 ml
Ajowan oil	2 ml
Alcohol (90% v/v)	A sufficient quantity

Method of preparation: Kalmegh is boiled with 1500 ml of water for half an hour and strained. Further, 1000 ml of water is added, boiled for half an hour and strained. The process is repeated until a total of 2000 ml of the extract is collected. The extract is mixed well and concentrated to 250 ml on a water bath. Ajowan oil and fennel oil are dissolved in 200 ml of alcohol (90% v/v), this alcoholic solution is added to the concentrated extract. The content of andrographolide is determined and enough Alcohol is added to produce a kalmegh liquid extract of the required strength.

Category: Bitter

Dose: 0.5 to 1 ml

KAOLIN POULTICE IP

Kaolin poultice contains 50.5% w/w of kaolin (limit: 48.0 to 53.0% w/w).

Ingredients	Official formula
Heavy kaolin, finely sifted, dried at 100 °C	527 g
Boric acid, finely sifted	45 g
Methyl salicylate	2 ml
Mentha oil	0.5 ml
Thymol	0.5 g
Glycerin	425 g

Method of preparation: Heavy kaolin and boric acid are mixed with Glycerin, heated at 120 °C for one hour, stirring occasionally. It is allowed to cool. Thymol previously dissolved in the Methyl salicylate is added followed by Mentha Oil. The resulting product is mixed thoroughly.

Category: Anti-inflammatory, Counter irritant.

KURCHI LIQUID EXTRACT IP

Kurchi liquid extract contains 1% w/v of the total alkaloids of kurchi (limit: 0.95 to 1.05% w/v).

Ingredients	Official formula
Kurchi, in fine powder	1000 g
Alcohol (60% v/v), sufficient quantity to produce 1000 ml	

Method of preparation: Kurchi is divided into three portions of 500, 300, 200 g. First portion (500 g) is mixed with sufficient alcohol (60% v/v) to render it evenly and distinctly damp. Then the moistened product is transferred to a suitable percolator. It is allowed to stand for 15 minutes, saturated with alcohol (60% v/v) and allowed to stand for about twenty-four hours. Percolation is started by using alcohol (60% v/v) as menstrum; the extract is collected in six separate, successive 250 ml portions numbering them in the same order in which they are received.

The second portion (300 g) of kurchi is moistened with a sufficient quantity of the first 250 ml portion of the percolate from the preceding lot of the drug. The rest of the first portion of the percolate is added and percolation process is started using as menstrum the other five percolates obtained from the first lot of the drugs. The percolate is collected in five successive of 250 ml portions, numbering them in the order in which they are received.

Similarly the third portion (200 g) of the kurchi is moistened with sufficient quantity of the first 250 ml portion of the percolate from the second lot of the drug and percolation is done using as menstrum the 250 ml portion of the percolate obtained from the second lot of the drug in the order received. The first 900 ml of the percolate is taken out. The percentage of the alkaloids in this percolate is determined by assay. To the rest of the liquid, sufficient alcohol (60% v/v) or a dilute extract of known alkaloid content is added to produce a kurchi liquid extract of the required strength. The product is set aside for not less than 24 h and filtered.

Category: Antiprotozoal

Dose: 8 to 16 ml.

STRONG LEAD SUBACETATE SOLUTION IP

Strong lead subacetate solution contains not less than 19 % w/w and not more than 21.5% w/w of total Pb; and has an alkalinity corresponding to not less than 10% w/w and not more than 12.5 % w/w of PbO.

Ingredients	*Official formula*
Lead acetate	250 g
Lead monoxide, in powder	175 g
Purified water, sufficient to produce 1000 ml	

Method of preparation: Lead acetate is dissolved in 750 ml of purified water; lead monoxide is added and kept aside for 48 h, shaking occasionally. The prepared solution is filtered and sufficient purified water is passed through the filter to produce required volume.

Category: Soothing astringent

DILUTE LEAD SUBACETATE SOLUTION IP

Ingredients	Official formula
Strong lead acetate solution	12.5 ml
Purified water, recently boiled and cooled, sufficient to produce 1000 ml	

Method of preparation: Strong lead acetate solution is mixed with purified water, recently boiled and cooled. Volume of the solution is made up to 1000 ml with purified water, recently boiled and cooled.

Category: Soothing astringent

LEPTAZOL INJECTION IP

Leptazol injection contains 10% w/v of leptazol (limit: 9.5 to 10.5% w/v).

Ingredients	Official formula
Leptazol	10 g
Sodium phosphate	0.25 g
Water for injection, sufficient to produce 100 ml	

Method of preparation: Leptazol and sodium phosphate are dissolved in 85 ml of water for injection; the reaction of the solution is adjusted to pH 7.8 by the addition of dilute hydrochloric acid or solution of sodium hydroxide. Sufficient water is added for injection to produce the required volume. The injection is filtered avoiding contact with metal. The above injection is sterilized by heating in an autoclave or by filtration, avoiding contact with metal.

Category: Central nervous system stimulant

Dose: By subcutaneous injection, 0.5 to 1 ml

LIGNOCAINE AND ADRENALINE INJECTION IP

Synonym: Lidocaine and adrenaline injection

Lignocaine and adrenaline Injection contains 2% w/v of lignocaine hydrochloride (limit: 1.9 to 2.10% w/v).

Ingredients	Official formula
Lignocaine hydrochloride	2 g
Sodium chloride	0.45 g
Adrenaline solution	100 ml
Sodium metabisulphate	0.1 g
Water for injection, sufficient quantity to produce 100 ml	

Method of preparation: Lignocaine hydrochloride, sodium chloride and sodium metabisulphate are dissolved in 80 ml of water for injection followed by addition of adrenaline solution and sufficient water for injection is added to produce the required volume. The prepared injection is sterilized by heating in an autoclave.

Category: Local anaesthetics

Dose: Dose should be determined by the prescriber

LIQUORICE COMPOUND POWDER IP

Ingredients	Official formula
Senna leaf, finely powdered	160 g
Liquorice, peeled, finely powdered	160 g
Fennel, finely powdered	80 g
Sulphur, sublimed	80 g
Sucrose, finely powdered	520 g

Method of preparation: All the constituents are mixed well together.

Category: Laxative

Dose: 4 to 8 g.

LIQUORICE LIQUID EXTRACT IP

Ingredients	Official formula
Liquorice, unpeeled, in coarse powder	1000 g
Chloroform water and alcohol (90% v/v) each of sufficient quantity	

Method of preparation: Liquorice is exhausted with chloroform water by percolation. The percolate is boiled for five minutes and kept aside for not less than 12 h. The clear liquid is decanted, the remainder is filtered and the two liquids are mixed well.

The extract is evaporated until the weight per ml of the liquid at 20 °C is 1.198 g. To this liquid, when cold, one fourth of its volume of alcohol (90 % v/v) is added. The product is allowed to stand for not less than four weeks and filtered.

Category: Demulcent

Dose: 2 to 4 ml

MAGNESIUM HYDROXIDE MIXTURE BPC

It consists of an aqueous suspension of hydrated magnesium oxide containing the equivalent of 7.9 % w/w of $Mg(OH)_2$.

Ingredients	Official formula
Light magnesium hydroxide	52.5 g
Sodium hydroxide	15 g
Magnesium sulphate	47.5 g
Chloroform water, double strength	500 ml
Purified water, freshly boiled and cooled to make up to 1000 ml	

Method of preparation: Sodium hydroxide is dissolved in 150 ml of purified water. Light magnesium oxide is added to form a smooth cream and sufficient purified water is added to produce 2500 ml. This suspension is poured into a solution prepared by dissolving required amount of magnesium sulphate in 2500 ml of water. Precipitate is allowed to subside and clear portion of liquid is removed. The residue is transferred to a calico strainer. The precipitate is washed with purified water until the washings give only a slight reaction for presence of sulphate. The washed precipitate is mixed with purified water and double-strength chloroform water is added. Sufficient purified water is added to the make up the volume up to 1000 ml.

MAGNESIUM SULPHATE PASTE BP

Synonym: Morison's paste

Ingredients	Official formula
Dried magnesium sulphate	q.s.
Phenol	0.5 g
Glycerol, previously heated at 120 °C for 1 h and cooled	55 g

Method of preparation: About 70 g of dried magnesium sulphate is dried for 1.5 h at 150 °C or 4 h at 130 °C. Then magnesium sulphate is cooled in desicators. 45 g of the dried material is mixed in a warm mortar with the phenol dissolved in glycerol.

Use: Edema and pain in boil and carbuncle.

COMPOUND MAGNESIUM TRISILICATE ORAL POWDER BP

Synonym: Compound magnesium trisilicate powder.

Ingredients	Official formula
Sodium potassium tartrate	7.5 g
Chalk, powder	250 g
Sodium bicarbonate	250 g
Heavy magnesium carbonate	250 g

Method of preparation: All the ingredients are mixed together properly.

Indication: Hyperacidity and peptic ulcer.

MEPHENESIN INJECTION IP

Mephenesin injection contains not less than 9.5% w/v and not more than 10.5% w/v of mephenesin $C_{10}H_{14}O_3$.

Ingredients	Official formula
Mephenesin	10 g
Alcohol	25 ml
Propylene Glycol	16 ml
Water for Injection, sufficient to produce 100 ml	

Method of preparation: Mephenesin is dissolved in a mixture of the alcohol, propylene glycol and sufficient water for Injection is added to produce 100 ml. The prepared injection is sterilized by filtration and distributed in ampoules or may be distributed in ampoules and sterilized by heating in an autoclave.

Category: Skeletal muscle relaxant

Dose: By intravenous infusion, 1 to 10 ml

OLEATED MERCURY IP

Oleated mercury contains the equivalent of 20 % w/w of yellow mercuric oxide (limit: 19.0 to 21.0 % w/w).

Ingredients	Official formula
Yellow mercuric oxide	200 g
Liquid paraffin	50 g
Oleic acid	750 g

Method of preparation: Mercuric oxide is triturated with liquid paraffin until it is thoroughly subdivided. Oleic acid is added and mixed thoroughly. The mixture is heated at 50 °C, triturating occasionally until combination is effected; when cool, a yellowish unctuous preparation is obtained.

Category: Anti-infective

Caution: Oleated mercury should not be dispensed if globules of mercury have separated

MERSALYL AND THEOPHYLLINE INJECTION IP

Synonym: Mersalyl injection.

Mersalyl and theophylline injection contains 10 % w/v of mersalyl, $C_{13}H_{16}O_6N \cdot NaHg$ (limit: 9.5 and 10.5 % w/v).

Ingredients	Official formula
Mersalyl acid	9.56 g
Theophylline	5 g
Sodium hydroxide	1 g or a sufficient quantity
Water for injection, sufficient to produce 100 ml	

Method of preparation: Mersalyl acid and theophylline is suspended in about 80 ml of water for injection, a 10 % w/v solution of sodium hydroxide in water for injection is added to the suspension with continuous stirring, until solution is affected. The reaction of the solution is adjusted to pH 8 by adding a further quantity of the solution of the sodium hydroxide and sufficient water for injection is added to produce 100 ml. The prepared injection is distributed in ampoules and sterilized by heating with a bactericide, using phenyl mercuric nitrate as the bactericide or may be sterilized by filtration and distributed in ampoules, contact of the solution with metal being avoided.

Category: Diuretic

Dose: By intramuscular injection, 0.5 to 2 ml (0.05 to 0.2) g of sodium salts of mersalyl acid and (0.025 to 0.1) g of theophylline on alternate days.

MORPHINE HYDROCHLORIDE SOLUTION IP

Morphine hydrochloride solution contains 1% w/v of morphine hydrochloride (limit: 0.95 to 1.05% w/v of $C_{17}H_{19}O_3N \cdot HCl \cdot 3H_2O$).

Ingredients	Official formula
Morphine hydrochloride	10 g
Dilute hydrochloric acid	20 ml
Alcohol (90 % v/v)	250 ml
Purified water, sufficient to produce 1000 ml	

Method of preparation: Alcohol (90% v/v) is diluted with an equal part of purified water followed by addition of dilute hydrochloric acid. Morphine hydrochloride is dissolved in the mixture and volume of the mixture is made up to 1000 ml with Purified water. The product is mixed well.

Category: Analgesic.

Dose: 0.3 to 2 ml.

Morphine hydrochloride solution contains 20 mg of morphine hydrochloride in 2 ml.

MORPHINE AND ATROPINE INJECTION IP

Morphine and atropine injection contains not less than 0.054% w/v and not more than 0.066% w/v of atropine sulphate, $(C_{17}H_{23}O_3N)_2 \cdot H_2SO_4 \cdot H_2O$ and not less than 0.90% w/v and more than 1.10% w/v of morphine sulphate, $(C_{17}H_{19}O_3N)_2 \cdot H_2SO_4 \cdot 5H_2O$.

Ingredients	Official formula
Atropine sulphate	0.06 g
Morphine sulphate	1 g
Water for injection, sufficient to produce 100 ml	

Method of preparation: Atropine sulphate and morphine sulphate is dissolved in part of water for injection and sufficient water for injection is added to produce 100 ml. The injection is sterilized by heating with a bactericide or by filtration.

Dose: By subcutaneous or intramuscular injection, 0.5 to 1 ml.

COMPOUND MYROBALAN POWDER IP

Ingredients	Official formula
Myrobalan (pulp only), in fine powder	100 g
Anise, in fine powder	100 g
Sucrose	100 g

Method of preparation: All the constituents are mixed together.

Category: Astringent.

Dose: 4 to 8 g.

SMALL MYROBALAN OINTMENT IP

Ingredients	Official formula
Small myrobalan ointment, in fine powder	20 g
Paraffin ointment	80 g

Method of preparation: Small myrobalan ointment, in fine powder, and paraffin ointment are mixed thoroughly by trituration.

Category: Astringent.

Dose: 2 to 4 g.

SMALL MYROBALAN AND OPIUM OINTMENT IP

Small myrobalan and opium ointment contains not less than 0.68 % w/w and not more than 0.83 % w/w of anhydrous morphine.

Ingredients	Official formula
Powdered opium, in fine powder	7.5 g
Small myrobalan ointment	92.5 g

Method of preparation: Powdered opium, in fine powder and small myrobalan ointment are mixed thoroughly by trituration.

Category: Astringent.

NUX VOMICA LIQUID EXTRACT IP

Nux vomica liquid extract contains 1.5% w/v of strychnine (limit: 1.425% w/v to 1.575% w/v).

Ingredients	Official formula
Nux vomica, in moderately coarse powder	1000 g
Alcohol (70% v/v) and alcohol (45% v/v) of each a sufficient quantity	

Method of preparation: Nux vomica is percolated with alcohol (70% v/v) until exhausted. Alcohol is recovered and the liquid is concentrated until it measures about 250 ml. To this liquid, while still hot, 25 g of hard paraffin is added, heated to 60°C and shaken vigorously. The product is allowed to cool, the solidified waxy layer is perforated and the liquid is poured off. 250 ml of alcohol (70% v/v) is added and filtered. The proportion of strychnine is determined in the liquid and to the remainder of liquid, sufficient alcohol (45% v/v) is added to produce a nux vomica liquid extract of the required strength. The resulting extract is kept aside for not less than 24 h and filtered.

Category: Bitter.

Dose: 0.06 to 0.2 ml.

Nux vomica liquid extract contains in 0.2 ml, 3 mg of Strychnine.

NUX VOMICA TINCTURE IP

Nux vomica tincture contains 0.125% w/v of strychnine (limit: 0.119 to 0.131% w/v).

Ingredients	Official formula
Nux vomica liquid extract	83.4 ml
Alcohol (45% v/v), sufficient to produce 1000 ml	

Method of preparation: Nux vomica liquid extract and alcohol (45% v/v) are mixed together and volume made up to 1000 ml with alcohol (45% v/v).

Category: Bitter

Dose: 0.6 to 2 ml

Nux vomica tincture contains in 2 ml, 2.5 mg of strychnine.

OPIUM TINCTURE IP

Synonym: Laudanum.

Opium tincture contains 1.0% w/v of morphine, calculated as anhydrous morphine (limit: 0.95% w/v to 1.05% w/v).

Ingredients	Official formula
Opium, sliced	200 g
Alcohol, (90% v/v)	a sufficient quantity
Purified water	a sufficient quantity

Method of preparation: 500 ml of boiling purified water is poured on to the opium and set aside for six hours. 500 ml of alcohol (90% v/v) is added and mixed thoroughly, set aside in a covered in a covered vessel for 24 h. The marc is strained and pressed, the liquids are mixed and set aside for not less than 24 hours; filtered.

The proportion of morphine is determined, calculated as anhydrous morphine, in the tincture so prepared using 40 ml. To the remainder of the liquid, sufficient of the mixture of equal volumes of alcohol (90% v/v) and purified water is added to produce an opium tincture of the required strength.

Category: Hypnotic, sedative

Dose: 0.3 to 2 ml

Opium tincture contains in 2 ml, 20 mg of anhydrous morphine.

CAMPHORATED OPIUM TINCTURE IP

Synonym: Compound camphor tincture

Camphorated opium tincture contains 0.05% w/v of morphine, calculated as anhydrous morphine (limit: 0.045% w/v to 0.055% w/v).

Ingredients	Official formula
Opium tincture	50 ml
Benzoic acid	5 g
Camphor	3 g
Anise oil	3 ml
Alcohol (60% v/v), sufficient to produce 1000 ml	

Method of preparation; Benzoic acid, camphor and anise oil is dissolved in 900 ml of alcohol (60% v/v). The opium tincture is added to the above, and sufficient alcohol (60% v/v) is added to produce the required volume; filtered.

Category: Hypnotic, sedative

Dose: 2 to 8 ml

Camphorated opium tincture contains 2 mg of anhydrous morphine in 4 ml of preparation.

ORAL REHYDRATION POWDER (ORS—WHO)

Ingredients	Official formula
Sodium chloride	3.5 g
Potassium chloride	1.5 g
Sodium bicarbonate	2.5 g
Anhydrous glucose	20 g
Transfer to a packet (One packet should be dissolved in 1000 ml purified water)	

Method of preparation: At first, potassium chloride is taken and then sodium bicarbonate is added. After mixing, sodium chloride is added and mixed. Now, anhydrous glucose is added in such a way that at each addition, the bulk quantity in the mortar or mixing tank doubles. The powder is mixed properly and transferred to a packet.

ORANGE TINCTURE IP

Ingredients	Official formula
Fresh orange peel, in thin slices	250 g
Alcohol (90% v/v)	1000 ml

Method of preparation: The product is prepared by maceration process.

Dose: 2 to 4 ml

PAEDIATRIC PARACETAMOL ELIXIR BPC

Ingredients	Official formula
Paracetamol	24 g
Chloroform spirit	20 ml
Concentrated raspberry juice	25 ml
Alcohol (95 %)	100 ml
Propylene glycol	100 ml
Invert syrup	275 ml
Amaranth solution	2 ml
Glycerol to make up the volume up to 1000 ml	

Method of preparation: A mixture of alcohol, chloroform spirit and propylene glycol is prepared. Paracetamol is dissolved in the above mixture. Concentrated raspberry juice is added with continuous mixing. Amarnath solution and sufficient glycerol is added to the mixture and stirred thoroughly.

Dose: Child's age up to 1 year: 5 ml

Child's age from 1 to 5 year: 10 ml

PAEDIARTIC PARACETAMOL SYRUP BP (125 mg/5 ml)

Ingredients	Official formula
Part 1	
Paracetamol	2.5 g
Polyethylene glycol 6000 (PEG 60000	10 g
Glycerin	2.5 g
Purified water	30 ml
Part 2	
Purified water	20 g
Sucrose	30 g
Sweetener	0.220 g
Sodium methyl paraben	0.150 g
Sodium propyl paraben	0.030 g

Ingredients	Official formula
Sodium benzoate	0.150 g
Citric acid monohydrate	0.070 g
Coloring agent	2.5 mg
Flavoring agent	0.25 ml

Method of preparation: Polyethylene glycol 6000 is heated at 50 °C and paracetamol is added to it. The solution is stirred for 30 minutes. Glycerin is heated at 50 °C and added to the paracetamol solution under continuous stirring for 20 minutes to form a transparent solution. Water is heated at 50 °C and the above solution is added to the water under continuous stirring.

Sucrose is weighed accurately and added to the hot water (65 °C) under continuous stirring till it dissolved. Citric acid monohydrate, sodium methyl paraben, sodium propyl paraben, sweetener and sodium benzoate are added to the water with continuous stirring for 10 minutes.

Then *Part 1* and *Part 2* are mixed till a clear solution is obtained. pH should be within 3.8–6.10; if not, add citric acid. Now color is added to the solution under continuous stirring. Volume is made up to 100 ml with water.

LIQUID PARAFFIN EMULSION IP

Liquid paraffin emulsion contains 50.0 % v/v of liquid paraffin (limit: 45.0 to 55.0 % v/v).

Ingredients	Official formula
Liquid paraffin	500 ml
Indian gum, in powder	125 g
Tragacanth, in powder	5 g
Sodium benzoate	5 g
Vanillin	0.5 g
Glycerin	125 ml
Chloroform	2.5 ml
Purified water, sufficient to produce 1000 ml	

Method of preparation: Liquid paraffin and chloroform is triturated with Indian gum, tragacanth and vanillin. 250 ml of purified water is added and triturated until a creamy emulsion is formed. Glycerin and sodium benzoate (which is dissolved in 50 ml of purified water) is added to the above emulsion. Sufficient purified water is added to produce 1000 ml and mixed well.

Category: Laxative.

Dose: 8 to 30 ml.

PARAFFIN OINTMENT IP

Ingredients	Official formula
White beeswax	20 g
Hard paraffin	30 g
Cetostearyl alcohol	50 g
White soft paraffin or yellow soft paraffin	900 g

Method of preparation: All the constituents are melted together, stirred, the source of heat is removed and stirring is continued until the mass reaches room temperature. When paraffin ointment is used in a white ointment, it should be prepared with white soft paraffin and when in a colored ointment, it should with yellow soft paraffin.

Category: Pharmaceutical aid

PENICILLIN EYE OINTMENT IP

Penicillin eye ointment contains not less than 90.0% of the stated number of units of benzyl penicillin.

Ingredients	Official formula
Benzyl penicillin	A sufficient quantity
Liquid paraffin	10 g
Wool fat	10 g
Yellow soft paraffin	80 g

Method of preparation: Wool fat, yellow soft paraffin and liquid paraffin are heated together, filtered while hot through a course filter paper placed in a heated funnel and sterilized by heating for a sufficient time to ensure that the entire matter is at 160 °C for at least one hour. The ointment is allowed to cool, benzyl penicillin is added and the mixture is triturated.

Category: Antibiotic.

Usual strength: 2000 units per g.

LIQUEFIED PHENOL IP

Synonym: Liquefied carbolic acid.

Liquefied phenol contains 80.0 % w/w of phenol (limit: 77.0 to 81.5 % w/w)

Ingredients	Official formula
Phenol	800 g
Purified water, sufficient to produce 1000 g	

Method of preparation: Phenol is warmed on a water bath until it is melted; purified water is added and mixed thoroughly.

Category: Disinfectant.

PHENOL GLYCERIN IP

Phenol glycerin contains phenol equivalent to 16.0 % w/w of C_6H_6O (limit: 15.0 to 16.5 % w/w).

Ingredients	Official formula
Phenol	160 g
Glycerin	840 g

Method of preparation: The two constituents are mixed together; warmed gently, if necessary, until solution is effected.

Category: Local analgesic, local antiseptic.

DILUTE PHOSPHORIC ACID IP

Ingredients	Official formula
Phosphoric acid	112 g
Purified water	888 g

Method of preparation: The two constituents are mixed well.

Category: Pharmaceutical aid

Dose: 0.3 to 4 ml

COMPOUND PICRORHIZA TINCTURE IP

Ingredients	Official formula
Picrorhiza, cut small and bruished	100 g
Dried orange peel, bruished	37.5 g
Cardamom, bruished	12.5 g
Alcohol (45% v/v)	1000 ml

Method of preparation: The product is prepared by the maceration process.

Category: Bitter

Dose: 2 to 4 ml

PIPERAZINE CITRATE ELIXIR IP

Piperazine citrate elixir contains not less than 14.0% and not more than 17.0% w/v of piperazine citrate (in anhydrous form) $3C_4H_{10}N_2.2C_6H_8O_7$.

Ingredients	Official formula
Piperazine citrate	180 g
Chloroform spirit	5 ml
Glycerin	100 ml
Orange oil	0.25 ml
Syrup	500 ml
Purified water, sufficient to produce 1000 ml	

Method of preparation: Piperazine citrate is dissolved in part of purified water. Orange oil, glycerin, syrup, chloroform spirit are added and sufficient purified water is added to produce the required volume.

Category: Antihelmintic

Dose: For threadworms, 4 to 15 ml daily, in divided doses; for roundworms, as a single dose up to 30 ml, according to the age of the patient.

POTASSIUM CHLORATE GARGLE BP

Ingredients	Official formula
Potassium chlorate	3.43 g
Solution of ferric chloride BP	3.10 ml
Glycerin	6.25 ml
Volume of water to make up to 100 ml.	

Method of preparation: Method of preparation: Potassium chlorate is dissolved in 50 ml of water. Solution of ferric chloride and glycerin is added to the above solution and mixed. Volume of the solution is made up to 100 ml with water.

PUNARNAVA LIQUID EXTRACT IP

Ingredients	Official formula
Punarnava, in coarse powder	1000 g
Alcohol (60% v/v)	Sufficient quantity
Purified water	Sufficient quantity

Method of preparation: The drug is exhausted by percolation process with alcohol (60% v/v) reserving the first 700 ml of the percolate. Alcohol is recovered from the remainder of the percolate by distillation and the residue is dissolved in the reserved portion. Sufficient purified water is added to make the volume up to 1000 ml. The extract is clarified by subsidence or by filtration.

Category: Diuretic

Dose: 2 to 8 ml

QUININE AND URETHANE INJECTION IP

Quinine and urethane injection contains not less than 11.9% w/w and not more than 13.1% w/w of quinine hydrochloride ($C_{20}H_{24}O_2N_2 \cdot HCl \cdot 2H_2O$) and not less than 5.65% w/w and not more than 6.85% w/w of urethane ($C_3H_7O_2N$).

Ingredients	Official formula
Quinine hydrochloride	12.5 g
Urethane	6.25 g
Water for injection, sufficient to produce 100 ml	

Method of preparation: Quinine hydrochloride and urethane are dissolved in water for injection by warming gently. The product is cooled; sufficient water for injection is added to produce the required volume and filtered. The injection is sterilized by heating in an autoclave or by filtration.

Category: Sclerosing agent

Dose: By intravenous injection, 0.5 to 5 ml

RESERPINE INJECTION IP

Reserpine injection contains not less than 0.24% w/v and not more than 0.26% w/v of reserpine, $C_{33}H_{40}O_9N_2$.

Ingredients	Official formula
Reserpine	0.25 g
Citric acid	0.2735 g
Benzyl alcohol	2 ml
Water for injection, sufficient to produce 100 ml	

Method of preparation: Reserpine and citric acid are placed in a stoppered container and 2 ml of the benzyl alcohol is added. Reserpine and citric acid are dissolved by warming gently on a water-bath. Sufficient water for injection is added to the solution to produce the required volume. The injection is sterilized by filtration.

Category: Hypotensive

Dose: By intramuscular injection, 0.25 to 1 mg

RHUBARB COMPOUND POWDER IP

Synonym: Gregory's powder

Ingredients	Official formula
Rhubarb, finely powdered	250 g
Light magnesium carbonate	325 g
Heavy magnesium carbonate	325 g
Ginger, finely powdered	100 g

Method of preparation: All the constituents are mixed together.

Category: Purgative

Dose: 0.6 to 4 g

SALICYLIC ACID OINTMENT IP

Salicylic acid ointment contains 2.0% w/w of salicylic acid (limit: 1.9 to 2.1% w/w).

Ingredients	Official formula
Salicylic acid, finely sifted	20 g
Wool alcohols ointment IP	980 g

Method of preparation: Wool alcohols ointment is melted; salicylic acid is added and stirred until cold.

Category: Local anti-infective

SODIUM SALICYLATE MIXTURE BP

Synonym: Sodium salicylate oral solution

Ingredients	Official formula
Sodium salicylate	50 g
Sodium metabisulphite	1 g
Concentrated orange peel infusion	50 ml
Double strength chloroform water	500 ml
Purified water sufficient to produce 1000 ml	

Indication: It is used as an analgesic-antipyretic in cases of pyrexia associated with bodyaches and in rheumatic fever.

SALICYLIC ACID LOTION BP

Ingredients	Official formula
Salicylic acid	20 g
Castor oil	10 g
Ethanol (96%), sufficient quantity to produce 1000 ml	

Method of preparation: The salicylic acid is dissolved in a portion of ethanol then castor oil and sufficient ethanol are added to produce 1000 ml.

Indication: As emollient and anti-microbial.

SHARK LIVER OIL WITH MALT EXTRACT IP

Shark liver oil with malt extract contains approximately 5 % w/w of shark liver oil and in 1 g not less than 300 International Units of vitamin A activity.

Ingredients	Official formula
Malt extract	950 g
Shark liver oil	50 g

Method of preparation: Malt extract and shark liver oil are mixed thoroughly, with the aid of gentle heat, if necessary.

Category: Nutrient

Dose: 4 to 16 ml

SIMPLE ELIXIR IP

Ingredients	Official formula
Orange tincture IP	75 ml
Syrup IP	400 ml
Chloroform water IP, qs ad	1000 ml

Method of preparation: Orange tincture is mixed with the syrup and sufficient chloroform water is added to produce the required volume. 25 g of purified talc is added and shaken, allowed to stand for few hours; shaking occasionally and filtered.

Category: Pharmaceutical aid.

Dose: 4 to 8 ml.

SIMPLE LINCTUS BPC

Ingredients	Official formula
Citric acid	25 g
Concentrated anise water	10 ml
Amaranth solution	15 ml
Chloroform spirit	60 ml
Syrup to make up the volume to 1000 ml	

Method of preparation: Citric acid is dissolved in a small amount of syrup. Anise water is mixed with chloroform. The two solutions are mixed together and stirred.

Dose: 5 ml

SIMPLE LINCTUS, PAEDIATRIC BPC

Ingredients	Official formula
Simple linctus	25 ml
Syrup to make up the volume to 100 ml	

Method of preparation: Simple linctus is mixed with syrup to prepare 100 ml.

Dose: 5 to 10 ml

SIMPLE OINTMENT IP

Ingredients	Official formula
Wool fat	50 g
Hard paraffin	50 g
Cetostearyl alcohol	50 g
White soft paraffin or yellow soft paraffin	850 g

Method of preparation: All the constituents are melted together and stirred until cold.

Category: Pharmaceutical aid

SOAP GLYCERIN SUPPOSITORIES USP

Ingredients	Official formula
Glycerin	91 g
Water	5 g
Sodium stearate	9 g

Method of preparation **(USP):** Glycerin is heated to 120 °C. Sodium stearate is dissolved in glycerin and water is added. Then the preparation is poured into mold and allowed to cool.

Method of preparation **(BPC) (Synonym:** *Suppositoria Glycerini Saponata***):** To make 10 rectal suppositories. Dissolve the sodium carbonate in the glycerin in a capsule on a water-bath; then add the stearic acid, and heat carefully until this is dissolved (table given below), and the escape of carbonic acid gas has ceased. Then pour the melted mass into suitable molds, remove the suppositories when they are cold, and wrap each in tin-foil. These suppositories should be freshly prepared when required.

Ingredients	Official formula
Glycerin	60 g
Sodium carbonate	3 g
Stearic acid	5 g

SOAP LINIMENT IP

Ingredients	Official formula
Soft soap	80 g
Camphor	40 g
Lemongrass oil	15 ml
Purified water	170 ml
Alcohol (90% v/v), sufficient to produce 1000 ml	

Method of preparation: Soft soap, camphor and lemongrass oil are dissolved in 600 ml of alcohol (90% v/v); purified water is added and sufficient alcohol (90% v/v) is added to produce required volume; set aside for a week and filtered.

Category: Detergent, mild local irritant.

COMPOUND SODIUM BICARBONATE TABLETS IP

Ingredients	Official formula
Sodium bicarbonate	320 mg
Mentha oil	0.004 ml

Method of preparation: Sodium bicarbonate is granulated by wet granulation method. To the dried granules mentha oil, previously dissolved in small volume of alcohol is added, mixed thoroughly and compressed into tablets.

Use: Antacid, electrolyte replenisher.

SODIUM CHLORIDE INJECTION IP

Synonym: Normal saline solution for injection.

Sodium chloride injection contains 0.9% w/v of sodium chloride (limit: 0.85–0.95% w/v).

Ingredients	Official formula
Sodium chloride	9 g
Water for injection, sufficient to produce 1000 ml	

Method of preparation: Sodium chloride is dissolved in water for injection. The solution is filtered and sterilized by heating in an autoclave or by filtration immediately.

Category: Electrolyte replenisher

COMPOUND SODIUM CHLORIDE INJECTION IP

Synonym: Ringer's injection

Compound sodium chloride solution contains in each 100 ml, not less than 0.82 g and not more than 0.90 g of sodium chloride, not less than 0.025 g and not more than 0.035 g of potassium chloride and not less than 0.30 g and not more than 0.36 g of calcium chloride hydrated, $CaCl_2 \cdot 6H_2O$.

Ingredients	Official formula
Sodium chloride	8.6 g
Potassium chloride	0.30 g
Calcium chloride hydrated	0.33 g
Water for injection, sufficient quantity to produce 1000 ml	

Method of preparation: All three salts are dissolved in water for injection and volume is made up to 1000 ml with water for injection. The solution is sterilized by heating in an autoclave or by filtration.

Category: Fluid and electrolyte replenisher.

COMPOUND SODIUM CHLORIDE SOLUTION IP

Synonym: Ringer's solution

Compound sodium chloride solution contains in each 100 ml, not less than 0.82 g and not more than 0.90 g of sodium chloride, not less than 0.025 g and not more than 0.035 g of potassium chloride and not less than 0.30 g and not more than 0.36 g of calcium chloride hydrated, $CaCl_2 \cdot 6H_2O$.

Ingredients	Official formula
Sodium chloride	8.6 g
Potassium chloride	0.30 g
Calcium chloride hydrated	0.33 g
Purified water, recently boiled, sufficient to produce 1000 ml	

Method of preparation: All three salts are dissolved in purified water (recently boiled) and volume is made up to 1000 ml with purified water (recently boiled). The solution is sterilized by heating in an autoclave or by filtration.

Category: Fluid and electrolyte replenisher.

SODIUM CITRATE ANTICOAGULANT INJECTION IP

Sodium citrate anticoagulant injection contains not less than 3.8% and not more than 4.2% w/v of $C_6H_5O_7Na_3 \cdot 2H_2O$.

Ingredients	Official formula
Sodium citrate	40 g
Water for Injection, sufficient to produce 1000 ml	

Method of preparation: Sodium citrate is dissolved in 900 ml of water for injection; filtered and sufficient water for injection is added to produce 1000 ml and immediately sterilized by heating in an autoclave or by filtration.

Category: Anticoagulant for plasma and for blood for fractionation.

COMPOUND SODIUM LACTATE INJECTION IP

Compound Sodium Lactate injection contains not less than 0.37% w/v and not more than 0.42% w/v of total Cl⁻, not less than 0.037% w/v and not more than 0.043% w/v of calcium chloride hydrated, $CaCl_2 \cdot 6H_2O$, and not less than 0.23% w/v and not more than 0.28% w/v of lactic acid, $C_3H_6O_3$.

Ingredients	Official formula
Sodium hydroxide	1.14 g
Dilute Hydrochloric acid	a sufficient quantity
Sodium chloride	6 g
Potassium chloride	0.4 g
Calcium chloride, hydrated	0.4 g
Water for injection, sufficient to produce 1000 ml	

Method of preparation: Sodium hydroxide is dissolved in 200 ml of water for injection; lactic acid is added and heated in an autoclave at 115 °C to 116 °C for one hour. The above solution is cooled and cautiously dilute hydrochloric acid (about 1 ml is normally required) is added until a few drops of the solution give orange color with solution of phenol red. Other ingredients are dissolved in 700 ml of water for injection, the two solutions are mixed and sufficient water for injection is added to produce 1000 ml. The resulting product is filtered and immediately sterilized by heating in an autoclave or by filtration.

Category: Fluid and electrolyte replenisher

STIBOPHEN INJECTION IP

Stibophen injection contains not less than 0.80% w/v and not more than 0.92% w/v of trivalent antimony.

Ingredients	Official formula
Stibophen	6.4 g
Sodium acid phosphate	0.25 g
Water for injection, sufficient to produce 100 ml	

Method of preparation: Stibophen and sodium acid phosphate are dissolved in about 80 ml of water for injection and sufficient water for injection is added to produce 100 ml. The injection is sterilized by heating in an autoclave or by filtration.

Category: Antiprotozoal

Dose: By intravenous injection, 1.5 to 5 ml

STRYCHNINE HYDROCHLORIDE SOLUTION IP

Synonym: Liquor strychninae hydrochloridi

Strychnine hydrochloride solution contains 1.0% w/v of $C_{21}H_{22}O_2N_2 \cdot HCl \cdot 2H_2O$ (limit: 0.95 to 1.05% w/v).

Ingredients	Official formula
Strychnine hydrochloride	10 g
Alcohol (90% v/v)	250 ml
Purified water, sufficient to produce 1000 ml	

Method of preparation: Alcohol (90% v/v) is mixed with an equal volume of purified water; strychnine hydrochloride is dissolved in the mixture and sufficient purified water is added to produce the required volume. The resulting solution is mixed well.

Category: Central stimulant

Dose: 0.2 to 0.8 ml

Strychnine hydrochloride solution contains 8 mg of strychnine hydrochloride in 0.8 ml.

SYRUP IP

Ingredients	Official formula
Sucrose	667 g
Purified water, sufficient to produce 1000 g	

Method of preparation: Sucrose is added to purified water and heated until dissolved with occasional stirring. Sufficient boiling purified water is added to produce 1000 g.

Category: Pharmaceutical aid

SULPHUR OINTMENT IP

Ingredients	Official formula
Sublimed sulphur, finely sifted	10 g
Simple ointment prepared with soft paraffin	90 g

Method of preparation: Sublimed sulphur is triturated with a small portion of ointment, and then gradually remaining part of the ointment is added and mixed thoroughly.

Use: It is used as a scabicide and mild antiseptic

DILUTE H_2SO_4 IP

Dilute sulphuric acid contains not less than 9.5% and not more than 10.5% w/w of H_2SO_4.

Ingredients	Official formula
Sulphuric acid	104 g
Purified water	896 g

Method of preparation: Sulphuric acid is added very gradually to the purified water and cooled.

Category: Pharmaceutical aid
Dose: 0.3 to 4 ml

TANNIC ACID GLYCERIN IP

Ingredients	Official formula
Sodium citrate	10 g
Dried sodium sulphite	2 g

Contd...

Ingredients	Official formula
Glycerin	788 g
Tannic acid	200 g

Method of preparation: Tannic acid, dried sodium sulphite and sodium citrateare rubbed in a porcelain dish with half of the glycerin until a smooth mixture is produced. Then the remainder glycerin is added and mixed well. The mixture is heated on a sand bath to a temperature between 115 °C and 120 °C with occasional stirring until solution is complete.

Category: Astringent

TALC DUSTING POWDER BP

Ingredients	Official formula
Starch, in powder	100 g
Purified talc	900 g

Method of preparation: The starch is triturated with the purified talc and the powder is passed through a sieve of suitable mesh size (250 μm).

The purified talc may be sterilized by dry heat, maintaining a temperature of not less than 160°C for not less than 1 h. Alternatively, the final product may be subjected to a sterilization procedure.

Indication: Absorb perspiration, and moisture after bathing.

TERPIN HYDRATE ELIXIR IP

Ingredients	Official formula
Terpin hydrate	50 g
Orange oil	0.2 ml
Glycerin	400 ml
Alcohol	425 ml
Syrup	100 ml
Purified water, sufficient quantity to make 1000 ml	

Method of preparation: Terpin hydrate is dissolved in the alcohol. Orange oil, syrup and glycerin are added and sufficient purified water is added to make up the volume up to 1000 ml.

The product is mixed well and filtered.

Category: Expectorant

Dose: 4 ml

TOLU SYRUP IP

Ingredients	Official formula
Tolu balsam	12.5 g
Sucrose	660 g
Purified water, sufficient to produce 1000 g	

Method of preparation: 400 ml of boiling purified water is added to the tolu balsam contained in a tarred vessel, the vessel is covered lightly and the contents is boiled gently for half an hour, stirring frequently. Purified water is added, if necessary, so that the contents of the vessel weigh 360 g. The solution is cooled and filtered. Sucrose is added, warmed on a water bath to dissolve and finally sufficient purified water is added to produce 1000 g.

Dose: 2 to 8 ml

TITANIUM DIOXIDE PASTE BP

Ingredients	Official formula
Titanium dioxide	200 g
Chlorocresol	1 g
Red ferric oxide, of commerce	20 g
Light kaolin or light kaolin, sterilized	100 g
Zinc oxide, finely sifted	250 g
Glycerol	150 g
Water, freshly boiled and cooled sufficient to produce	1000 g

Method of preparation: The light kaolin or light kaolin (natural), titanium dioxide and zinc oxide are mixed to form a homogenous powder. The chlorocresol is dissolved in the glycerol, the water is added and the solution is triturated gradually with the mixed powders to form a smooth paste.

Use: Protective against sun burn

TURPENTINE LINIMENT IP

Turpentine liniment yields, on distillation in steam, not less than 63.0% v/w and not more than 70.0% v/w of volatile oil and camphor.

Ingredients	Official formula
Soft soap	90 g
Camphor	50 g
Turpentine oil (freshly rectified)	650 ml
Purified water, sufficient to produce 1000 ml	

Method of preparation: Soft soap is mixed with 100 ml of purified water. A solution of camphor is made in the freshly rectified turpentine oil. Gradually the camphor solution is added to the soap mixture with trituration until a thick creamy emulsion is formed. Sufficient purified water is added to produce the required volume and mixed well.

Category: Counterirritant, rubefacient

URGINEA TINCTURE IP

Ingredients	Official formula
Urginea, bruished	100 g
Alcohol (60% v/v)	1000 ml

Method of preparation: The product is prepared by maceration process.

Category: Cardiotonic and expectorant

Dose: 0.3 to 2 ml

URGINEA VINEGAR IP

Ingredients	Official formula
Urginea, bruished	100 g
Dilute acetic acid	1000 ml

Method of preparation: Urginea is macerated with dilute acetic acid in a closed vessel for 7 days, with occasional agitation. The liquid is drained off and the marc is pressed. The two liquids is mixed and heated to boiling. The product is set aside for not less than seven days and filtered.

Category: Cardiotonic and expectorant

Dose: 0.6 to 2 ml

URGINEA SYRUP IP

Ingredients	Official formula
Urginea vinegar	450 ml
Sucrose	800 g
Purified water, sufficient to produce 1000 ml	

Method of preparation: Sucrose is dissolved in the urginea vinegar by the aid of gentle heat, strained and when cold, sufficient purified water is added to produce the required volume.

Category: Cardiotonic and expectorant

Dose: 2 to 4 ml

AMMONIATED VALERIAN TINCTURE IP

Ammoniated valerian tincture contains 0.875% w/v of NH_3 (limit: 0.70 to 1.05% w/v).

Ingredients	Official formula
Valerian, in moderately coarse powder	200 g
Nutmeg oil	3 ml
Lemon oil	2 ml
Dilute ammonia solution	100 ml
Alcohol (60% v/v)	900 ml

Method of preparation: All the liquid ingredients are mixed together. Maceration process is carried out to prepare the tincture.

Category: Sedative

Dose: 2 to 4 ml

VASAKA LIQUID EXTRACT IP

Ingredients	Official formula
Vasaka, in no. 40 powder	1000 g
Alcohol (40% v/v)	a sufficient quantity

Method of preparation: The drug is exhausted by percolation process, reserving the first 800 ml of the percolate. Alcohol is recovered from the remainder of the percolate by distillation and the residue is evaporated to the consistence of a soft extract. This part is dissolved in the reserved portion. Alcohol (40% v/v) is added to produce 1000 ml.

Category: Expectorant

Dose: 1 to 2 ml

VASAKA SYRUP IP

Ingredients	Official formula
Vasaka liquid extract	500 ml
Glycerin	100 ml
Syrup, sufficient to produce 1000 ml	

Method of preparation: Vasaka liquid extract is mixed with glycerin and enough syrup is added to produce 1000 ml. The extract is mixed thoroughly.

Category: Expectorant

Dose: 2 to 4 ml

WOOL ALCOHOLS OINTMENT IP

Ingredients	Official formula
Wool alcohols	60 g
Hard paraffin	240 g
White soft paraffin or yellow soft paraffin	100 g
Liquid paraffin	600 g

Method of preparation: All the constituents are melted together, stirred until cold.

In preparing this ointment, the proportions of hard paraffin, soft paraffin and liquid paraffin may be varied and the liquid paraffin may be replaced wholly or partly by light liquid paraffin in order to produce wool alcohols ointment having suitable properties.

When wool alcohols ointment is used in a white ointment, it should be prepared with white soft paraffin and when used in a colored ointment, it should be prepared with yellow soft paraffin.

Category: Emollient, pharmaceutical aid.

HYDROUS OINTMENT IP

Synonym: Oily cream

Ingredients	Official formula
Wool alcohols ointment	500 g
Purified water	500 ml

Method of preparation: Wool alcohols ointment is melted and the purified water is added to the above gradually with constant stirring. The product is mixed vigorously until a smooth cream is obtained, stirred until room temperature is attained.

When hydrous ointment is used in a white ointment, it should be prepared from wool alcohols ointment made with white soft paraffin; when used in a colored ointment, it should be prepared from wool alcohol ointment made with yellow soft paraffin.

Category: Pharmaceutical aid

HYDROUS WOOL FAT IP

Synonym: Lanolin

Ingredients	Official formula
Wool fat	700 g
Purified water	300 ml

Method of preparation: Wool fat is melted and purified water is added gradually with constant stirring, till the mass is homogeneous.

Category: Pharmaceutical aid.

ZINC OXIDE COMPOUND PASTE IP

Synonym: Zinc paste

Zinc oxide compound paste contains 25.0% w/w of zinc oxide (limit: 23.5 to 26.5% w/w).

Ingredients	Official formula
Zinc oxide, finely sifted	250 g
Starch, finely sifted	250 g
White soft paraffin	500 g

Method of preparation: White soft paraffin is melted; zinc oxide and starch are incorporated to it. The product is stirred until cold.

Category: Astringent, pharmaceutical aid

HYDROUS ZINC OXIDE OINTMENT IP

Hydrous zinc oxide ointment contains 15.0% w/w of ZnO (limit: 14.0 to 15.5% w/w).

Ingredients	Official formula
Zinc oxide, finely sifted	150 g
Hydrous ointment	850 g

Method of preparation: Zinc oxide is triturated with a portion of the hydrous ointment until smooth; the remainder is added gradually and mixed thoroughly.

Category: Astringent, pharmaceutical aid

ZINC OXIDE OINTMENT IP

Synonym: Zinc ointment.

Zinc oxide ointment contains 15.0% w/w of ZnO (limit: 14.0 to 15.5% w/w).

Ingredients	Official formula
Zinc oxide, finely sifted	150 g
Simple ointment	850 g

Method of preparation: Zinc oxide is triturated with a portion of the simple ointment until smooth; the remainder is added gradually and mixed thoroughly.

Category: Astringent, pharmaceutical aid

ZINC ICHTHAMMOL CREAM IP

Ingredients	Official formula
Ichthammol	50 g
Cetostearyl alcohol	30 g
Wool fat	100 g
Zinc cream, sufficient to produce	1000 g

Method of preparation: Wool fat and cetostearyl alcohol are melted together with the aid of gentle heat, the mixture is triturated with 800 g of zinc cream until smooth, ichthammol is incorporated, sufficient zinc cream is added to produce 1000 g and mixed.

Use: Protective cream in eczema, psoriasis

ZINC AND SALICYLIC ACID PASTE BP

Synonym: Lassar's paste.

Ingredients	Official formula
Zinc oxide, finely sifted	240 g
Salicylic acid, finely sifted	20 g
Starch, finely sifted	240 g
White soft paraffin	500 g

Method of preparation: White soft paraffin is melted, zinc oxide, salicylic and starch are incorporated and stirred until cold.

Use: Eczema

ZINC UNDECYLENATE OINTMENT IP

Zinc undecylenate ointment contains 20% w/w of zinc undecylenate (limit: 18.5 to 21.5% w/w of $C_{22}H_{38}O_4Zn$).

Ingredients	Official formula
Zinc undecylenate	200 g
Undecylenic ointment	50 g
Emulsifying ointment	750 g

Method of preparation: Emulsifying ointment is melted. Zinc undecylenate and undecylenic acid are added to the ointment. The product is stirred until room temperature is attained.

Category: Fungistatic ointment

WHITEFIELD'S OINTMENT IP

Synonym: Compound benzoic acid ointment, benzoic acid and salicylic acid ointment.

Ingredients	Official formula
Benzoic acid, in fine powder	6 g
Salicylic acid, in fine powder	3 g
Emulsifying ointment	91 g

Method of preparation: Benzoic acid and salicylic acid are triturated with a portion of emulsifying ointment until smooth and then the remainder of the emulsifying ointment is incorporated.

Indication: Fungal infections

Appendices

Appendices

Appendix 1
Physiological Units

| Table A1.1 | Blood, serum and plasma |

Blood (B), Serum (S), Plasma (P)	Values
Blood pH normal range	7.35–7.45
O_2 partial pressure in arterial blood	75–100 mmHg
O_2 partial pressure in venous blood	35–45 mmHg
O_2 content	16.5–20.0 ml/dl
O_2 saturation in arterial blood	96%–98%
O_2 saturation in venous blood	70%–80%
CO_2 partial pressure in arterial blood	35–45 mmHg
CO_2 content in arterial blood	47–51 ml/dl
CO_2 partial pressure in venous blood	41–51 mmHg
CO_2 content in venous blood	51–55 ml/dl
Osmolarity of body fluids	280–300 mOsm/L
Serum creatinine	0.5–1.5 mg/dl
Serum sodium ion	136–145 mmoles/L or mEq/L
Serum potassium ion	3.5–5.0 mmoles/L or mEq/L
Serum calcium ion	4.5–5.5 mEq/L
Serum chloride ion	96–106 mmoles/L or mEq/L
Serum glucose (fasting)	65–110 mg/dl
Serum urea	8–20 mg/dl
Serum phosphate	1.8–2.6 mEq/L
Cholesterol, total	150–250 mg/dl
LDL fraction	80–150mg/dl
HDL fraction	30–60 mg/dl
VLDL fraction	20–40 mg/dl
Serum albumin	3.2–5.6 g/dl
Serum bicarbonate	22–26 mEq/L
RBC count (males)	$4.5–6.2 \times 10^6$ cells/microlitre
Hematocrit (males)	40%–52%

Contd...

Blood (B), Serum (S), Plasma (P)	Values
Hemoglobin (males)	14–17 g/dl
RBC (females)	4–5.5 × 10^6 cells/microlitre
Hematocrit (females)	37%–47%
Hemoglobin (females)	12–16 g/dl
WBC count	4–11 × 10^3 cells/microlitre
Platelets	200–500 × 10^3 platelets/microlitre
Heamoglobin average O_2	
(carrying capacity)	1.34 ml/g of Hb
Bilirubin, total	0.2–1 mg/dl
Direct	<0.4 mg/dl
Indirect	<0.6 mg/dl
Glucose, fasting (B)	70–100 mg/dl
Hemoglobin (B)	
Male	14–16 mg/dl
Female	13–15 mg/dl
Phospholipids	150–200 mg/dl
Triglycerides, fasting	75–150 mg/dl
Urea (B)	15–40 mg/dl
Urea nitrogen (B), BUN	8–20 mg/dl
Uric acid	
Male	4–8 mg/dl
Female	3.5–6 mg/dl

Table A1.2 Proteins

Total proteins	6.4–8.3 g/dl
Albumin (S)	3.5–5.5 g/dl
Fibrinogen (P)	0.2–0.6 g/dl
Globulin (S)	2–3.6 g/dl
Transferrin	200–300 mg/dl

Table A1.3 Enzymes

Name of Enzyme	Values
Acid phosphatase (ACP) or 2.5–12 IU/L or 10–100 nkat.	0.5–4 King-Armstrong U/dl
Alanine transaminase (ALT, SGPT)	3–40 IU/L or 40–250 nkat
Aspartate transaminase (AST, SGOT)	4–45 IU/L or 50–320 nkat
Alkaline phosphatase (ALP)	In adults, 3–13 King-Armstrong (KA) U/dl
Amylase	8–180 Somogyi U/dl or 2.5–5.5 μkat

Contd...

Name of Enzyme	Values
Aspartate transaminase (AST, SGOT)	4–45 IU/L or 50–320 nkat
Creatine kinase	10–50 IU/L
Cholinesterase	2–10 IU/L
Ceruloplasmin	20–50 mg/dl
γ-Glutamyl transpeptidase	5–40 IU/L
Lactate dehydrogenase	50–200 IU/L or 1–5 µkat
Lipase	0.2–1.5 IU/L
Ceruloplasmin	20–50 mg/dl
Glucose 6-phosphate Dehydrogenase in RBC	120–260 IU/10^{12} RBC
Isocitrate dehydrogenase	1–4 IU/L

Table A1.4 Hormones

Name of Hormone	Values
Growth hormone (hGH) (S)	In adults, up to 300 ng/dl
	In children, up to 500 ng /dl
Thyroid stimulating hormone (THS) (P)	2 U/ml
Follicle stimulating hormone (FSH) (S)	Perpuberal, 2–12 mIU/ml
	Adult men, 1–15 mIU/ml
	Adult women, 1–30 mIU/ml
	Postmenopausal, 30–200 mIU/ml
Luteinizing hormone (LH) (S)	Perpuberal, 2–12 mIU/ml
	Adult men, 1–15 mIU/ml
	Adult women, < 30 mIU/ml
	Postmenopausal, > 30 mIU/ml
Adrenocorticotropic hormone (ACTH) (P)	3 ng/dl
Prolactin (S)	0–20 ng/ml
Somatomedin C (P)	0.4–2 U/ml
Antidiuretic hormone (P)	Serum osmolality 285 mOsm/kg, 0–2 pg/ml
Cortisol	5–15 µg/dl
11-deoxycorticosterone (P)	0.006 mg/dl
Estradiol	
Female	10–45 ng/dl
Male	<5 ng/dl
Insulin	6–25 µU/ml
Testosterone	
Adult male	300–800 ng/dl
Adult female	25–50 ng/dl
Thyroid stimulating hormone	5–10 µU/dl
Triiodothyronine	110–180 ng/dl
Thyroxin	5–12 µg/dl

Table A1.5 Inorganic substance

Name of Inorganic Substances	Values
Ammonia (P)	80–100 µg/dl
Anion gap (calculated)	10–18 mEq/L
Bicarbonate	22–26 mEq/L
Calcium	9–11 mg/dl
Chloride	96–106 mEq/L
Copper	100–200 µg/dl
Iodine	4–10 µg/dl
Iron	50–150 µg/dl
Magnesium	1.5–2.0 mEq/L
Phosphorus	3–4.5 mg/dl
Potassium	3.5–5 mEq/L
Sodium	135–145 mEq/L

Table A1.6 Cardiac function

Cardiac output (CO)	4.0–8.0 L/min
Central venous pressure	2–7 mmHg
Diastolic pressure (average, systemic)	60–90 mmHg
Systolic pressure (average, systemic)	90–140 mmHg
Mean arterial pressure (average, systemic)	70–105 mmHg
Diastolic pressure (average, pulmonary)	4–13 mmHg
Systolic pressure (average, pulmonary)	17–32 mmHg
Mean arterial pressure (average, pulmonary)	9–19 mmHg

Table A1.7 Cerebrospinal fluid

Appearance	Clear and colorless
Specific gravity	1.003–1.008
Albumin	8–30 mg/dl
Chloride	120–130 mg/dl
Gamma globulin	1.3–4.7 mg/100 ml, 4.3–12.3 % of total protein
Glucose	50–85 mg/dl
Protein, total	15–40 mg/dl
IgG	2–6 mg/dl
Cells	
Adults	0–5 mononuclears/µl
Infants	0–20 mononuclears/ µl

Table A1.8 Semen

Sperm count	60–150 million/ml
Leucocytes	Occasional or absent
Morphology	80–90% normal forms
Motility	80% or more mobile
pH	7.2–8
Volume	2–6 ml
Specific gravity	1.028
Osmolarity	296 mOsm/kg
Protein	32.9–77.4 mg/ml
Mucoproteins	9 mg/ml
Lipids	1.67–2.06 mg/ml
Na^+	100–133 mmol/L
K^+	17–27.4 mmol/L
Ca^{2+}	5.3–7.2 mmol/L
Mg^{2+}	5.3 mmol/L
Cl^-	28.3–57.3 mmol/L
Organic phosphates	10 mg/ml
Inositol	3.3 mmol/L
Fructose	12 mmol/L
Pyruvate	1.4–7 mmol/L
Citrate	5–76 mmol/L
Urea	12 mmol/L
Creatine	1.3 mmol/L
Choline	6.8 mmol/L
Phosphorylcholine	2.86–3.8 mg/ml

Table A1.9 Stool

Bulk	100–200 g daily (upto 350 g with high vegetable diet)
Dry matter	23–32 g daily (upto 75 g in high vegetable diet)
Fat total	17.5% of dry matter
Fatty acid combined as soap	4.6% of dry matter
Free fatty acid	5.6% of dry matter
Neutral fat	7.3% of dry matter (42% of total fat)
Nitrogen excretion	less than 1.7 g/day
Urobilinogen	40–280 mg/day
pH	5.9–8.5
Bilirubin	5–20 mg/day

Table A1.10	Urine
Volume	1–1.5 L
Specific gravity	1.003–1.030
pH	4.5–6
Color	Normally straw color
Osmolarity	1200 mOsm/L
Acetone	Negative
Erythrocytes	0–130,000/24 h
Leucocytes	0–650,000/24 h
Aldosterone	2–26 µg/24 h
Alpha amino nitrogen	64–199 mg/24 h
Ammonia	40 mmols/day
Amylase	Up to 400 U/h
Bilirubin	Negative
Catecholamine, total	<100 µg/24 h
Calcium	
Low calcium diet	less than 150 mg/24 h
Usual diet	less than 250 mg/24 h
Chloride	200 mmols/day
Creatine	0–100 mg/day
Creatinine	10 mmols/day
17-hydroxycorticoids	
Male	4–12 mg/24 h
Female	4–8 mg/24 h
17-keto steroids	
Male	10–20 mg/24 h
Female	5–15 mg/24 h
Oxalic acid	20–40 mg/day
Phosphorus	0.5–1.5 g/day
Potassium	50 mmols/day
Phosphate	25 mmols/day
Specific gravity	1.003–1.030
Sodium	200 mmols/day
Sulfate	50 mmols/day
Titrable acidity	20–40 mEq/24 h
Urea	400 mmols/day
Uric acid	4 mmols/day
Urobilinogen	0–3.5 mg/day

Table A1.11　Vitamins

Vitamin A(S)	30–95 µg/dl
Thiamine (S)	0.07–0.88 r/100 ml
Vitamin D	25-Hydroxycholecalciferol 10–55 ng/ml; 1, 25-dihydroxy-cholecalciferol 24–65 pg/ml
Riboflavin(P)	1–19 µg/L
Vitamin B_6(P)	5–24 ng/ml
Vitamin B12(S)	>150–590 pmol/L
Ascorbic acid	
Plasma	0.2–2.0 mg/dl
W.B.C	25–40 mg/100 ml

Table A1.12　pH of important biological fluids

Name of the Biological Fluid	pH
Pancreatic juice	7.5–8.0
Blood plasma	7.35–7.45
Cerebrospinal fluid	7.2–7.4
Tears	7.2–7.4
Interstitial fluid	7.2–7.4
Human milk	7.2–7.4
Saliva	6.4–7.0
Intracellular fluid	6.5–6.9
Gastric juice	1.5–3.0
Urine	5.0–7.5

Table A1.13　Daily water loss

Site	Vol/Day (ml)
Skin	500
Expired Air	350
Urine	1500
Feces	150
Total	**2500**

Table A1.14　Amniotic fluid

Creatinine	> 2.0 mg/dl
Lecithin/sphingomyelin (L/S ratio)	> 2.0 indicates maturity

Appendix 2
Physical Units

List of physical quantities

Physical Quantities	Relation with Other Quantities	Dimensional Formula	SI Coherent Derived Unit
Area	Length × breadth	$L \times L = L^2 = [M^0 L^2 T^0]$	m^2
Volume	Length × breadth × height	$L \times L \times L = [M^0 L^3 T^0]$	m^3
Density	Mass/volume	$M/L^3 = [ML^{-3}T^0]$	$kg \cdot m^{-3}$
Speed or velocity	Distance/time	$L/T = [M^0 LT^{-1}]$	$m \cdot s^{-1}$
Acceleration	Change in velocity/time	$LT^{-1}/T = LT^{-2} = [M^0 LT^{-2}]$	$m \cdot s^{-2}$
Momentum	Mass × velocity	$M \times LT^{-1} = [MLT^{-1}]$	$kg\ m \cdot s^{-1}$
Force	Mass × acceleration	$M \times LT^{-2} = [MLT^{-2}]$	N
Work	Force × distance	$MLT^{-2} \times L = [ML^2T^{-2}]$	J
Energy	Amount of work	$[ML^2T^{-2}]$	J
Power	Work/time	$ML^2T^{-2}/T = [ML^2T^{-3}]$	W
Pressure	Force/area	$ML^1T^{-2}/L^2 = [ML^{-1}T^{-2}]$	Pa or $N \cdot m^{-2}$
Moment of force or torque	Force × perpendicular distance	$MLT^{-2} \times L = [ML^2T^{-2}]$	$N \cdot m$
Gravitational constant 'g'	Force × (distance)^2/mass × mass	$MLT^{-2}L^2/M \times M = [M^{-1}L^3T^{-2}]$	$N \cdot m^2 \cdot kg^{-2}$
Impulse of a force	Force × time	$MLT^{-2} \times T = [MLT^{-1}]$	$N \cdot s$
Stress	Force/area	$MLT^{-2}/L^2 = [ML^{-1}T^{-2}]$	$N \cdot m^{-2}$
Strain	Change in dimension/ original dimension	$[M^0L^0T^0]$ (Dimensionless)	–
Coefficient of elasticity	Stress/strain	$ML^{-1}T^{-2} = [ML^{-1}T^{-2}]$	$N \cdot m^{-2}$
Surface tension	Force/length	$MLT^{-2}/L = MT^{-2} = [ML^0T^{-2}]$	$N \cdot m^{-1}$

Contd...

196

Physical Quantities	Relation with Other Quantities	Dimensional Formula	SI Coherent Derived Unit
Surface energy	Work/area	$ML^2T^{-2}/L^2 = MT^{-2} = [ML^0T^{-2}]$	$J \cdot m^{-2}$
Coefficient of viscosity	Force × distance/area × velocity	$MLT^{-2} \times L/L^2 \times LT^{-1} = [ML^{-1}T^{-1}]$	$N \cdot s \cdot m^{-2}$ or Pas
Angle	Arc/radius	$L/L = 1 = [M^0L^0T^0]$ (dimensionless)	Rad
Angular velocity	Angle/time	$1/T = T^{-1} = [M^0L^0T^{-1}]$	$Rad \cdot s^{-1}$
Angular acceleration	Angular velocity/time	$T^{-1}/T = T^{-2} = [M^0L^0T^{-2}]$	$Rad \cdot s^{-2}$
Moment of inertia	Mass × (distance)²	$ML^2 = [ML^2T^0]$	$kg \cdot m^2$
Radius of gyration	Distance	$L = [M^0LT^0]$	M
Angular momentum	Mass × velocity × radius	$M \times LT^{-1} \times L = [ML^2T^{-1}]$	$kg \cdot m^2 \cdot s^{-1}$
Time period	Time	$T = [M^0L^0T]$	s
Frequency	1/time period	$1/T = T^{-1} = [M^0L^0T^{-1}]$	s^{-1} or Hz
Planck's Constant 'h'	E/ν = Energy/frequency	$ML^2T^{-2}/T^{-1} = [ML^2T^{-1}]$	$J \cdot s$
Relative density	Density of substance/ density of water at 4 °C	$ML^{-3}/ML^{-3} = 1 = [M^0L^0T^0]$ (dimensionless)	–
Velocity gradient	Velocity/distance	$LT^{-1}/L = T^{-1} = [M^0L^0T^{-1}]$	s^{-1}
Pressure gradient	Pressure/distance	$ML^{-1}T^{-2}/L = [ML^{-2}T^{-2}]$	$Pa \cdot m^{-1}$
Force constant	Force/displacement	$MLT^{-2}/L = MT^{-2} = [ML^0T^{-2}]$	$N \cdot m^{-1}$

Table A2.2 **List of thermal quantities**

Thermal Quantities	Relation with Other Quantities	Dimensional Formula	SI Coherent Derived Unit
Heat or enthalpy	Energy	$[ML^2T^{-2}]$	J
Specific heat	Heat/mass × temperature	$ML^2T^{-2}/M.K = [M^0L^2T^{-2}K^{-1}]$	$J \cdot kg^{-1} \cdot K^{-1}$
Latent heat	Heat/mass	$ML^2T^{-2}/M = [M^0L^2T^{-2}]$	$J \cdot kg^{-1}$
Thermal conductivity	Heat × distance/area × temp × time	$ML^2T^{-2}.L/L^2.K.T = [MLT^{-3}K^{-1}]$	$J \cdot s^{-1} \cdot m^{-1} \cdot K^{-1}$
Entropy	Heat/temperature	$ML^2T^{-2}/K = [ML^2T^{-2}K^{-1}]$	$J \cdot K^{-1}$
Universal gas constant	Pressure × volume/amount × temperature	$[ML^2T^{-2}K^{-1}]$	$J \cdot mol^{-1} \cdot K^{-1}$
Boltzmann's constant	Energy/temperature	$ML^2T^{-2}/K = [ML^2T^{-2}K]$	$J \cdot K^{-1}$
Stefan-Boltzmann's constant	Energy/area × time × (temp.)⁴	$ML^0T^{-3}K^{-4}$	$J \cdot s^{-1} \cdot m^{-2} \cdot K^{-4}$
Solar constant	Energy/area× time	ML^2T^{-2}/L^2T	$J \cdot s^{-1} \cdot m^{-2}$

Table A2.3 List of electrical quantities

Electrical Quantities	Relation with Other Quantities	Dimensional Formula	SI Unit
Electric charge	Time × current	$T \times A = [M^0L^0TA]$	C (coulomb)
Electrical potential	Work/charge	$ML^2T^{-2}/TA = [ML^2T^{-3}A^{-1}]$	V(volt)
Resistance	Potential difference/ current	$ML^2T^{-3}A^{-1}/A = [ML^2T^{-3}A^{-2}]$	Ω(ohm)
Capacitance	Charge/potential difference	$TA/ML^2T^{-3}A^{-1} = [M^{-1}L^{-2}T^4A^2]$	F(farad)
Inductance	Emf/current/time	$ML^2T^{-3}A^{-1}/AT^{-1} = [ML^2T^{-2}A^{-2}]$	H(henry)
Permittivity of free space	$\varepsilon_0 = q_1q_2/Fr^2$	$AT \times AT/MLT^{-2}L^2 = [M^{-1}L^{-3}T^4A^2]$	F/m
Relatve permittivity or dielectric constant	$\kappa = \varepsilon_0/\varepsilon$	A pure ratio = $[M^0L^0T^0]$ (Dimensionless)	–
Intensity of electric field	$E = F/q = $ Force/charge	$MLT^{-2}/AT = [MLT^{-3}A^{-1}]$	$N \cdot C^{-1}$ or $V \cdot m^{-1}$
Conductance	$C = 1/$resistance	$1/ML^2T^{-3}A^{-2} = [M^{-1}L^{-2}T^3A^2]$	Ω^{-1} or mho
Specfic resistance or resistivity	$\sigma = RA/l$	$ML^2T^{-3}A^{-2}L^2/L = [ML^3T^{-3}A^{-2}]$	$\Omega \cdot m$
Specific con- ductance or con- ductivity		$1/M^{-1}L^{-3}T^3A^2 = [M^{-1}L^{-3}T^3A^2]$	$\Omega^{-1} \cdot m^{-1}$
Electric dipole moment	$q \times 2l$	$AT \times L = [M^0LTA]$	$C \cdot m$

Table A2.4 List of magnetic quantities

Magnetic Quantities	Relation with Other Quantities	Dimensional Formula	SI Coherent Derived Unit
Magnetic field	$B = F/qvsinr$	$MLT^{-2}/AT \times LT^{-1} \times 1 = [M^0T^{-2}A^{-1}]$	T (tesla)
Magnetic flux	$\phi = BA$	$MT^{-2}A^{-1}L^2 = [ML^2T^{-2}A^{-1}]$	Wb (weber)
Permeability of free space	$\pi_0 = 4\pi r.F/I_1I_2/$	$L \times MLT^{-2}/A^2 \times L = [MLT^{-2}A^{-2}]$	–
Pole strength	Magnetic moment/ magnetic length	$AL^2/L = [M^0LT^0A]$	$A \cdot m$

Table A2.5 Some useful conversion factors

Some Useful Conversion Factors
1 nanometre $= 10^{-9}\,m$
1 picometre $= 10^{-12}\,m$
1 litre $= 10^{-3}\,m^3$
1 calorie $= 4.184\,J$
1 electron volt (eV) $= 1.6022 \times 10^{-19}\,J$
1 angstrom (Å) $= 10^{-10}\,m$

Name	Symbol	Value in SI units
Nautical mile	–	1 nautical mile = 1852 m
Knot	–	1 nautical mile per hour = (1852/3600) m/s
Angstrom	Å	$1\ \text{Å} = 10^{-10}$ m
Barn	B	$10^{-28}\,\text{m}^2$
Bar	bar	1 bar $=10^5$ Pa
Curie	Ci	$1\ \text{Ci} = 3.7 \times 10^{10}\,\text{Bq}$
Roentgen	R	$1\ \text{R} = 2.58 \times 10^{-4}\,\text{C/kg}$
Rad	rad	$1\ \text{rad} = 10^{-2}\,\text{Gy}$
Rem	rem	$1\ \text{rem} = 10^{-2}\,\text{Sv}$
Erg	erg	$1\ \text{erg} = 10^{-7}\,\text{J}$
Dyne	dyn	$1\ \text{dyn} = 10^{-5}\,\text{N}$
Poise	P	$1\ \text{P} = 0.1\ \text{Pa} \cdot \text{s}$
Stokes	St	$1\ \text{St} = 1\ \text{cm}^2/\text{s} = 10^{-4}\,\text{m}^2/\text{s}$
Gauss	Gs, G	$10^{-4}\,\text{T}$
Maxwell	Mx	$1\ \text{Mx} = 10^{-8}\,\text{Wb}$
Torr	Torr	$1\ \text{Torr} = (101325/760)$ Pa
Standard atmosphere	atm	1 atm = 101325 Pa
Fermi	Fermi	$1\ \text{fermi} = 10^{-13}\,\text{m}$
Photometric carat	metric carat	$1\ \text{metric carat} = 2 \times 10^{-4}\,\text{kg}$

To Convert From	To	Multiply by
acre	square metre (m^2)	4.046873×10^3
acre foot	cubic metre (m^3)	1.233489×10^3
ampere hour $(\text{A} \cdot \text{h})$	coulomb (C)	3.6×10^3
atmosphere, standard (atm)	pascal (Pa)	1.01325×10^5
bar (bar)	pascal (Pa)	10^5
barrel [for petroleum, 42 gallons (U.S.)](bbl)	cubic metre (m^3)	1.589873×10^{-1}
barrel [for petroleum, 42 gallons (U.S.)](bbl)	litre (L)	1.589873×10^2
British thermal unit (BTU)	joule (J)	$1.05505585262 \times 10^3$
British thermal unit foot per hour square foot degree Fahrenheit $[\text{BTU} \cdot \text{ft}/(\text{h} \cdot \text{ft}^2 \cdot {}^\circ\text{F})]$	watt per metre kelvin $[\text{W}/(\text{m} \cdot \text{K})]$	1.730735
British thermal unit inch per hour square foot degree Fahrenheit $[\text{BTU} \cdot \text{in}/(\text{h} \cdot \text{ft}^2 \cdot {}^\circ\text{F})]$	watt per metre kelvin $[\text{W}/(\text{m} \cdot \text{K})]$	1.442279×10^{-1}
British thermal unit inch per second square foot degree Fahrenheit $[\text{BTU} \cdot \text{in}/(\text{s} \cdot \text{ft}^2 \cdot {}^\circ\text{F})]$	watt per metre kelvin $[\text{W}/(\text{m} \cdot \text{K})]$	5.192204×10^2

Contd...

To Convert From	To	Multiply by
British thermal unit per cubic foot (Btu/ft³)	meter (J/m³)	3.725895×10^4
British thermal unit per degree Fahrenheit (Btu/°F)	joule per kelvin (J/K)	1.899101×10^3
British thermal unit per hour (Btu/h)	watt (W)	2.930711×10^{-1}
British thermal unit per hour square foot degree Fahrenheit [Btu/ (h · ft² · °F)]	watt per square metre kelvin [W/(m² · K)]	5.678263
British thermal unit per pound (Btu/lb)	joule per kilogram (J/kg)	2.326×10^3
British thermal unit per pound degree Fahrenheit [Btu /(lb· °F)]	joule per kilogram kelvin [(J/(kg · K)]	4.1868 c
British thermal unit per second (Btu/s)	watt (W)	1.055056×10^3
British thermal unit per second square foot degree Fahrenheit [Btu /(s · ft².°F)]	watt per square metre kelvin [W/(m²· K)]	2.044175×10^4
calorie(cal)	joule(J)	4.1868
calorie per gram (cal/g)	joule per kilogram (J/kg)	4.1868×10^3
calorie per second (cal/s)	watt (W)	4.184
centimetre of mercury (0 °C)	pascal (Pa)	1.33322×10^3
centipoise (cP)	pascal second (Pa·s)	10^{-3}
centistokes (cSt)	meter squared per second (m²/s)	10^{-6}
carat, metric	kilogram (kg)	2×10^{-4}
cubic foot (ft³)	cubic metre (m³)	2.831685×10^{-2}
cubic foot per minute (ft³/min)	cubic metre per second (m³/s)	4.719474×10^{-4}
cubic foot per minute (ft³/min)	litre per second (L/s)	4.719474×10^{-1}
cubic foot per second (ft³/s)	cubic metre per second (m³/s)	2.831685×10^{-2}
cubic inch (in³)	cubic metre (m³)	1.683706×10^{-5}
cubic mile (mi³)	cubic metre (m³)	4.168182×10^9
cubic yard (yd³)	cubic metre (m³)	7.645549×10^{-1}
curie (Ci)	becquerel (Bq)	3.7×10^{10}
debye (D)	coulomb metre (C · m)	3.335641×10^{-30}

Contd...

To Convert From	To	Multiply by
degree Celsius (temperature) (°C)	kelvin (K)	$T/K = t/°C + 273.15$
degree Fahrenheit (temperature) (°F)	degree Celsius (°C)	$t/°C = (t/°F - 32)/1.8$
degree Fahrenheit (temperature) (°F)	kelvin (K)	$T/K = (t/°F + 459.67)/1.8$
degree Rankine (°R)	kelvin (K)	$T / K = (T/°R) / 1.8$
dyne (dyn)	newton (N)	10^{-5}
dyne centimetre (dyn·cm)	newton metre (N · m)	10^{-7}
electronvolt (eV)	joule (J)	1.602176×10^{-19}
erg (erg)	joule (J)	10^{-7}
erg per second (erg/s)	watt (W)	10^{-7}
erg per square centimetre second [erg/(cm² · s)]	watt per square metre (W/m²)	10^{-3}
faraday (based on carbon 12)	coulomb (C)	9.648534×10^4
fluid ounce (U.S.) (fl oz)	millilitre (ml)	2.957353×10^1
foot (ft)	metre (m)	3.048×10^{-1}
foot per second (ft/s)	metre per second (m/s)	3.048×10^{-1}
franklin (Fr)	coulomb (C)	3.335641×10^{-10}
gal (Gal)	metre per second squared (m/s²)	10^{-2}
gallon (U.S.) (gal)	litre (L)	3.785421
gallon (U.S.) per horse-power hour [gal/(hp · h)]	cubic metre per joule (m³/J)	1.410089×10^{-9}
gamma (γ)	tesla (T)	10^{-9}
gauss (Gs, G)	tesla (T)	10^{-4}
grain (gr)	milligram (mg)	6.479891×10
grain per gallon (U.S.) (gr/gal)	kilogram per cubic metre (kg/m³)	1.711806×10^{-2}
hectare (ha)	square metre (m²)	10^4
horsepower (metric)	watt (W)	7.354988×10^2
Inch(in)	metre (m)	2.54×10^{-2}
Inch(in)	centimetre (cm)	2.54
kilowatt hour (kW · h)	joule (J)	3.6×10^6
Litre (L)	cubic metre (m³)	10^{-3}
maxwell (Mx)	weber (Wb)	10^{-8}
Mho	siemens (S)	1
millimeter of mercury, conventional (mmHg)	pascal (Pa)	1.333224×10^2
ounce (avoirdupois) (oz)	kilogram (kg)	2.834952×10^{-2}
ounce (U.S. fluid) (fl oz)	millilitre (ml)	2.957353×10
ounce (avoirdupois) per gallon [Canadian and U.K. (Imperial)] (oz/gal)	gram per litre (g/L)	6.236023

Contd...

To Convert From	To	Multiply by
ounce (avoirdupois) per gallon(U.S.)(oz/gal)	gram per litre (g/L)	7.489152
parsec (pc)	metre (m)	3.085678×10^{16}
phot (ph)	lux (lx)	1×10^4
pint (U.S. dry) (dry pt)	litre (L)	5.506105
pint (U.S. liquid) (liqpt)	litre (L)	4.731765
poise (P)	pascal second (Pa·s)	1×10^{-1}
pound (avoirdupois) (lb)	kilogram (kg)	4.535924×10^{-1}
pound (troy or apothecary) (lb)	kilogram (kg)	3.732417×10^{-1}
pound-force (lbf)	newton (N)	4.448222
pound-force foot (lbf · ft)	newton metre (N · m)	1.355818
pound-force per square foot (lbf/ft²)	pascal (Pa)	4.788026
pound per cubic foot (lb/ft³)	kilogram per cubic metre (kg/m³)	1.601846×10^1
pound per horsepower hour [lb/(hp · h)]	kilogram per joule (kg/J)	1.689659×10^{-7}
quart (U.S. dry) (dry qt)	litre (L)	1.101221
quart (U.S. liquid) (liqqt)	litre (L)	9.463529
rad (absorbed dose) (rad)	gray (Gy)	10^{-2}
roentgen (R)	coulomb per kilogram (C/kg)	2.58×10^{-4}
rpm (revolution per minute) (r/min)	radian per second (rad/s)	1.047198×10
slug (slug)	kilogram (kg)	1.459390×10
stokes (St)	meter squared per second (m²/s)	10^{-4}
ton, metric (t)	kilogram (kg)	10^3
year (365 days)	second (s)	3.1536×10^7

To Convert From	To	Multiply by
angstrom	nanometre (nm)	0.1
fathom	metre(m)	1.828804
foot (ft)	metre (m)	0.3048
inch (in)	millimetre (mm)	25.4
microinch (iin)	micrometre (μm)	0.0254
mil (0.001 inch)	millimetre(mm)	0.0254
mil (0.001 inch)	micrometre (μm)	25.4
yard (yd)	metre (m)	0.9144
nautical mile	kilometre (km)	1.852
pica	millimetre (mm)	4.2175

To Convert From	To	Multiply by
acre-foot	cubic metre(m^3)	1233.489
cubic yard	cubic metre (m^3)	0.764555
cubic foot	cubic metre (m^3)	0.02831685
cubic foot	litre (L)	28.31685
Bushel	cubic metre (m^3)	0.03523907

To Convert From	To	Multiply by
Standard acceleration of gravity (g_n)	metre per second squared ($m \cdot s^{-2}$)	9.80665
foot per second squared	metre per second squared ($m \cdot s^{-2}$)	0.3048
inch per second squared	metre per second squared ($m \cdot s^{-2}$)	0.0254

To Convert From	To	Multiply by
gallon per minute	litre per second (L/s)	0.0630902
gallon per day	litre per day (L/d)	3.785412
cubic yard per minute	litre per second (L/s)	12.74258
cubic foot per minute	cubic metre per second (m^3/s)	0.0004719474
cubic foot per minute	litre per second (L/s)	0.4719474
cubic foot per second	cubic metre per second (m^3/s)	0.02831685

To Convert From	To	Multiply by
acre	hectare(ha)	0.4046873
square foot	square metre (m^2)	0.09290304
square yard	square metre (m^2)	0.83612736
square mile	square kilometre (km^2)	2.589988
square inch	square centimetre (cm^2)	6.4516
square inch	square millimetre (mm^2)	645.16

Table A2.6 Examples of units contrary to SI units

Quantities	Name of Unit	Symbol	Value in SI Units
Length	angstrom	A	10^{-10} m = 10^{-1} nm
	Inch	In	2.54×10^{-2} m
	micron	μm	10^{-6} m
	Mile	mile	1.6×10 m
Volume	Litre	L	10^{-3} m^3
Force	dyne	dyn	10^{-5} N
Pressure	Atmosphere	atm	101325 N m^{-2}
	Torr	Torr	(101325/760) N m^{-2}
	conventional milli-meter of mercury	mm Hg	13.5951×980.665 $\times 10^{-2}$ N m^{-2}
	Pascal	Pa	N m^2
	bar	bar	10^5 pa or 10^5 N m^{-2}
Mass energy	Pound	lb	0.453592 kg
	erg	erg	10^{-7} J
	Cal	Cal	4.184 J
	electron volt	eV	1.6021×10^{-19} J

Table A2.7 Physical and chemical quantities

Quantities	Symbol
Absorbance	A
Equilibrium constant	K
Michaelis constant	Km
Relative molecular mass	Mr
Retardation factor	RF
Specific rotation	[α]
Sedimentation coefficient	S

Table A2.8 Absorption coefficient of gases at 293 °K

Solvent	H_2	He	N_2	O_2	CO_2	H_2S	NH_3	HCL
Water	0.017	0.009	0.015	0.028	0.88	2.68	710	442
Benzene	0.066	0.018	0.104	0.163	–	–	–	–
Alcohol	0.08	0.028	0.13	0.143	0.177	3	–	–

Table A2.9 Effect of temperature on solubility of gases

GAS	0 °C	20 °C	60 °C
N_2	0.003 g	0.002 g	0.001 g
O_2	0.007 g	0.004 g	0.002 g
CO_2	0.377 g	0.2 g	0.07 g
NH_3	0.983 g	0.574 g	0.225 g

Table A2.10	Molal elevation constants of solvents (ebullioscopic constant)	
Solvent	Boiling point(in °C)	K_b(in °C · kg · mol⁻¹)
Water	100	0.512
Acetic acid	118.1	3.07
Carbon tetrachloride	76.8	4.95
Benezene	80.1	2.53
Carbon disulfide	46.2	2.37
Phenol	181.75	3.04
Napthalene	217.9	5.8

Table A2.11	Molal depression constants (cryoscopic constants) of solvents	
Solvent	Freezing point (in °C)	K_f(in °C · kg · mol⁻¹)
Aniline	–5.96	–5.87
Benzene	5.5	–5.12
Carbon disulphide	–111.5	–3.83
Chloroform	–63.5	–4.90
Ethanol	–114.6	–1.99
Phenol	43.0	–7.27

Table A 2.12	Specific conductance of a few substances at 298 °K
Substance	k (ohm⁻¹cm⁻¹)
Glass	1×10^{-14}
Graphite	1.2×10^{3}
Iron metal	1.0×10^{5}
Silver metal	5.0×10^{5}
Teflon	1.0×10^{-16}
0.1 M NaCl	9.2×10^{-2}
0.01 M NaCl	1.2×10^{-3}
0.1 M HCl	3.5×10^{-4}
0.001 M CH₃COOH	4×10^{-5}
0.01 M CH₃COOH	1.6×10^{-4}
Pure water	1×10^{-6}

Table A2.13	Equivalent conductance of electrolytes at 298 °K				
Concentration (g equiv/L)	*HCl*	*NaOH*	*NaCl*	*CH_3COOH*	*NH_4OH*
0.1	391.32	–	106.74	5.2	3.6
0.05	399.09	–	111.06	7.4	11.3
0.002	407.24	–	115.76	11.6	34
0.01	412	238	118.51	16.2	46.9
0.005	415.8	240.8	120.65	22.8	–
0.001	421.36	244.7	123.74	48.6	–
0.0005	422.74	245.6	124.5	–	–
(infinite dilution)	426.16	247.8	126.45	–	–

Table A2.14	Equivalent conductance at infinite dilution [cm^2 (g equiv)$^{-1}$ Ohm^{-1}] of some pairs of electrolytes	
Electrolyte	*Λ_0*	*Difference*
KNO_3 and KIO_3	144.96 and 117.56 respectively	27.40
$NaNO_3$ and $NaIO_3$	121.55 and 94.15 respectively	27.40
KF and NaF	129.21 and 105.79 respectively	23.42
KCl and NaCl	149.86 and 126.45 respectively	23.41
KNO_3 and $NaNO_3$	144.96 and 121.55 respectively	23.41
KBr and NaBr	151.92 and 128.51 respectively	23.41
NaCl and NaF	126.45 and 105.79 respectively	20.66
KBr and KCl	151.92 and149.86 respectively	2.06
NaBr and NaCl	128.51 and 126.45 respectively	2.06
LiBr and LiCl	117.09 and 115.03 respectively	2.06

Table A2.15	Conversion of units	
To Convert From	*To*	*Multiply by*
Mass and related derived units		
kilogram	pound (avoirdupois)	2.2046
kilogram	gram	1000
pound (avoirdupois)	gram	453.59
ton (metric)	kilogram	1000
ton (metric)	pound (avoirdupois)	2204.6
gram per cu.cm	pound per cu.ft	62.43
pound per cu.ft	gram per cu.cm	0.016018
pound per cu.ft	kilogram per cu.m	16.018
Length and related derived units		
centimetre	angstrom units	10^8
micron	angstrom units	10^4
centimetre	micron	10^4
metre	centimetre	100

Contd...

To Convert From	To	Multiply by
metre	millimetre	1000
foot	metre	0.3048
metre	foot	3.2808
inch	centimetre	2.54
foot per minute	cm per second	0.508
Time		
hour	minutes	60
minute	seconds	60
Area		
sq.in	sq.cm	6.452
sq.cm	sq.ft	0.0010764
sq.ft	sq.m	0.0929
Volume and related derived units		
cubic metre	litres	1000
cubic foot	gallons	7.481
gallons	cu.m	0.003785
us gallons	imperial gallons	0.8327
gallons	litres	3.785
gallons per min	cu.ft per sec	0.002228
gallons	cu.in	231
Pressure		
cm of Hg at 0 °C	ft of water at 39.1 °F	0.446
cm of Hg at 0 °C	pound per sq.in	0.19837
gram per sq.in.	pound per sq.in	0.014223
kg per sq.in	pound per sq.in	14.223
atmosphere	mm hg at 32 °F	760
atmosphere	ft. of water at 39.1 °F	33.9
atmosphere	gram per sq.cm	1033.3
atmosphere	pound per sq.in	14.698
bar	pascal	10^5
atmosphere	pascal	1.01325×10^5
bar	pound per sq.in	14.504
Viscosity		
centipoise	poise	0.01
centipoise	lb/hr.ft	2.42
centipoise	lb/sec.ft	0.000672
english unit	centipoise	1488
Heat		
centigrade heat unit	Btu	1.8
kilowatt hour	Btu	3414
kilowatt	Horse power	1.341
Btu	Calories	252.16
Btu	foot-pound	777.9
Btu/lb. °F	cal/g °C	1
Btu/hr.ft². °F	kg . cal/hr. m²°C	4.88
g.cal/hr.cm².°C/cm	Btu/hr . ft² . °F/in	0.8064

Contd...

To Convert From	To	Multiply by
Energy		
foot-pound	kilowatt hour	3.766×10^{-7}
foot pound/sec	kilowatt	0.0013558
horsepower (British)	Btu/hr	2545
horsepower (British)	ft lb/sec	550
horsepower (British)	horsepower (metric)	1.0139
watts	Btu/h	3.413
kilowatt hour	Btu	3413
ton (refrigeration)	Btu/h	12000

Table A2.16 Capsule number and its approximate capacity

Empty capsule size

Capsule size	000	00E	00	0E	0	1	2	3	4	5
Empty capsule weight (gelatin)										
Average weight(mg)	158	143	136	107	105	79	63	50	40	30
Tolerance	±10	±10	±7	±7	±6	±5	±4	±3	±3	±2
Empty volume capsule capacity (ml)	1.37	1.00	0.90	0.78	0.68	0.48	0.36	0.27	0.20	0.13
Empty capsule weight capacity by formulation density (mg)										
0.6 g/ml	822	600	540	468	408	288	216	162	120	78
0.8 g/ml	1096	800	720	624	544	384	288	216	160	1-4
1.0 g/ml	1370	1000	900	780	680	480	360	270	200	130
1.2 g/ml	1644	1200	1080	936	816	576	432	324	240	156
Empty capsule overall closed length (mm)	26.1	25.3	23.4	23.5	21.6	19.4	17.6	15.7	14.7	11.1
Tolerance for overall length	±0.3	±0.3	±0.3	±0.3	±0.3	±0.3	±0.3	±0.3	±0.3	±0.4

Table A2.17 Surface tension of liquids

Liquids	Surface tension (dyn/cm)
Methanol	22.70 (20 °C)
Propyl alcohol	22.89 (30 °C)
Benzene	28.20 (25 °C)
Toluene	28.40 (20 °C)
Xylene	27.5
Carbon tetrachloride	25.5
Xylene	27.5
Diethyl ether	17.1 (20 °C)
1,2-Dichloro ethane	33.30 (20 °C)

Contd...

Liquids	Surface tension (dyn/cm)
1,2,3-Tribromo propane	45.40 (20 °C)
1,4-Dioxane	33 (20 °C)
1-Decanol	28.50 (20 °C)
1-nitro propane	29.40 (20 °C)
1-Octanol	27.60 (20 °C)
Benzylalcohol	39 (20 °C)
Benzylbenzoate	45.95 (20 °C)
Bromobenzene	36.50 (20 °C)
Bromoform	41.50 (20 °C)
Chloroform	27.50 (20 °C)
Cyclohexane	24.95 (20 °C)
Dichloromethane	26.50 (20 °C)
Diethylene glycol	44.80 (20 °C)
Dipropylene glycol	33.90 (20 °C)
Ethanol	22.10 (20 °C)
Ethylbenzene	29.20 (20 °C)
Ethylene glycol	47.70 (20 °C)
Isoamylchloride	23.50 (20 °C)
Isobutylchloride	21.90 (20 °C)
m-Nitrotoluene	41.40 (20 °C)
Mercury	425.41 (20 °C)
Methyl ethyl ketone	24.60 (20 °C)
N,N-dimethyl formamide (DMF)	37.10 (20 °C)
N-methyl-2-pyrrolidone	40.79 (20 °C)
n-Decane (DEC)	23.83 (20 °C)
n-Octane (OCT)	21.62 (20 °C)
n-Hexane (HEX)	18.43 (20 °C)
n-Tetradecane (TDEC)	26.56 (20 °C)
n-Undecane	24.66 (20 °C)
n-Butylbenzene	29.23 (20 °C)
n-Propylbenzene	28.99 (20 °C)
Nitroethane	31.90 (20 °C)
Nitrobenzene	43.90 (20 °C)
Nitromethane	36.80 (20 °C)
o-Nitrotoluene	41.50 (20 °C)
Perfluorohexane	11.91 (20 °C)
Phenylisothiocyanate	41.50 (20 °C)
Polyethylen glycol 200 (PEG)	43.50 (20 °C)
Polydimethylsiloxane (Baysilone M5)	19 (20 °C)
Pyridine	38 (20 °C)
Pyrrol	36.60 (20 °C)
Tetrahydrofuran	26.40 (20 °C)
Water	72.80 (20 °C)
o-Xylene	30.10 (20 °C)
α-Bromonaphthalene	44.40 (20 °C)

Table A2.18 Gold number values of some important colloids

Protective Colloid	Gold Number
Gelatin	0.005–0.01
Albumin	0.15–0.25
Acacia	0.1–0.2
Sodium oleate	1–5
Tragacanth	2
Potato starch	20–25
Haemoglobin	0.03–0.07
Sodium caseinate	0.01

Table A2.19 Concentration expressions

Expression	Symbol	Definition
Molarity	M, C	Moles (gram molecular weights) of solute in 1 litre of solution
Normality	N	Gram equivalent weights of solute in 1 L of solution
Molality	M	Moles of solute in 1000 g of solvent
Mole fraction	X, N	Ratio of the moles of one constituent (e.g. the solute) of a solution to the total moles of all constituents (solute and solvent)
Mole percent		Moles of one constituent in 100 moles of the solution; mole percent is obtained by multiplying mole fraction by 100
Percent by weight	% w/w	Gram of solute in 100 g of solution
Percent by volume	% v/v	Millilitres of solute in 100 ml of solution
Percent weight-in-volume	% w/v	Gram of solute in 100 ml of solution
Milligram percent	–	Milligram of solute in 100 ml of solution

Appendix 3
Different Types of Pipette

Pipettes are basically classified into two categories:

1. *Pipette TD:* These pipettes are calibrated to deliver. These pipettes should be drained in vertical position and then touched against the wall of vessel to drain the tips.

2. *Pipette TC:* Pipettes calibrated to contain are used for viscous liquid such as syrup. This type of pipette should be washed after draining the liquid and washing should be added to measuring portion. These pipettes are known as blow out pipettes. Liquid should be expelled out using a rubber bulb.

Based on nature, pipettes can be divided into the following categories:

1. *Graduated pipette:* Graduated pipette consist of glass tube of uniform bore with graduation marks evenly space along the length the tube to indicate different calibrated volume. They require a source of vacuum. These pipettes are used for delivery of specific amount of liquid. These pipettes are divided into two categories.

   (a) *Mohr pipette:* These pipettes are calibrated between two graduation marks on the stem of glass tube. In this type of pipette, there is no need to drain out liquid completely.

   (b) *Serological pipette:* This type of pipette has graduation mark down to the tip of the pipette.

2. *Volumetric pipette or bulb pipette:* These pipettes have a large bulb with a long narrow portion above with a single mark. It is calibrated for single volume. Volume of solution can be measured precisely with these pipettes.

3. *Pasteur pipette:* These pipettes are used to transfer small amounts of liquids. They are generally not graduated or calibrated for any particular volume. The bulb is separate from the pipette body. These pipettes are used as droppers, eye droppers and chemical droppers.

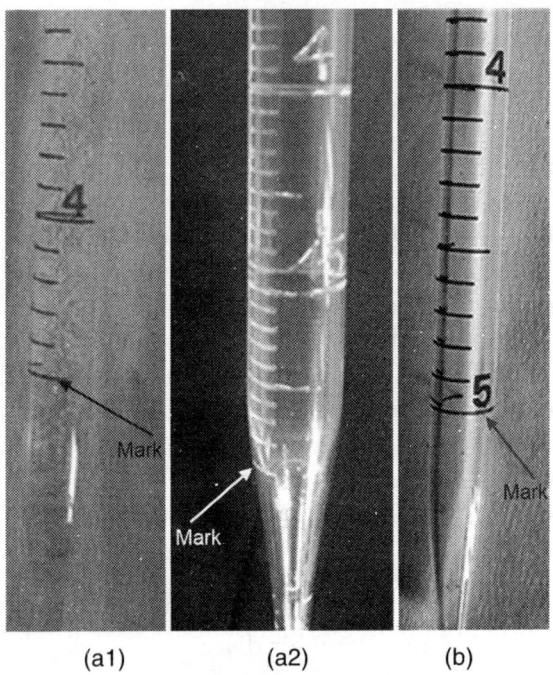

(a1)   (a2)   (b)

Figure A3.1: (a) Serological pipette (b) Mohr pipette

4. *Beral pipette:* These pipettes are similar to Pasteur pipettes but are made from a single piece of plastic and their bulb can serve as the liquid-holding chamber.

5. *Van Slyke pipette:* It is a graduated pipette and discovered by Donald Dexter Van Slyke.

6. *Ostwald-Folin pipette:* It is a specialized pipette used in measuring viscous solution such as whole blood.

7. *Single channel pipette:*These are developed pipetting tool. These pipettes are based on piston. They have only one channel to deliver the liquid as glass pipette. They can be operated manually or electronically. Manually operated single channel pipette are already discussed in air displacement and positive displacement pipette. In case of Electronic pipette, uptake and dispensing are controlled by a microprocessor installed in the pipette rather than manually plunger button. They are very accurate in delivering exact quantity of liquid. They can be programmed as per need of the user. In recent years electronic pipette undergoes many advances. Easy user interface, ability to control aspiration and dispensing of liquid makes electronic pipette more versatile. These pipettes can be used to transfer different type of liquid with different viscosities. With electronic pipette, it is possible to mix two mix liquids in the tip with repeated movement of the piston of the pipette.

8. *Air displacement pipette:* These pipettes are operated by piston-driven air displacement. A vacuum is generated by the vertical travel of a metal or ceramic piston within an airtight sleeve. As the piston moves upward, a partial vacuum is created in the space left vacant by the piston. The liquid around the tip moves into this vacuum. This liquid can be transferred as necessary. These pipettes are precise and accurate. They are extremely accurate with aqueous solution. As they rely on air displacement, this may result inaccuracies due to changing environment, particularly temperature and user technique.

9. *Positive displacement pipette:* These pipettes are based on disposable piston and capillary system which is in direct contact with the sample. When the piston is moved upward, sample is drawn into the capillary. Positive-displacement pipettes provide high accuracy and precision

when pipetting aqueous solution. These pipettes are recommended for use with viscous, dense, volatile and corrosive solutions.

10. *Multichannel pipette:* They have multiple channels to deliver liquid. They have the same as single channel pipette but they are applied for high applications such as ELISA test. They are also available in manual and electronic format.

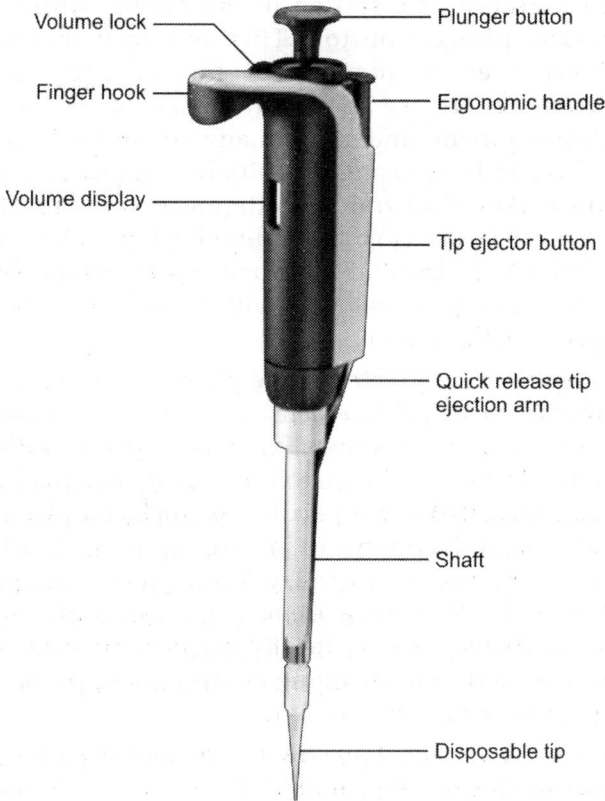

Figure A3.2: Single channel pipette

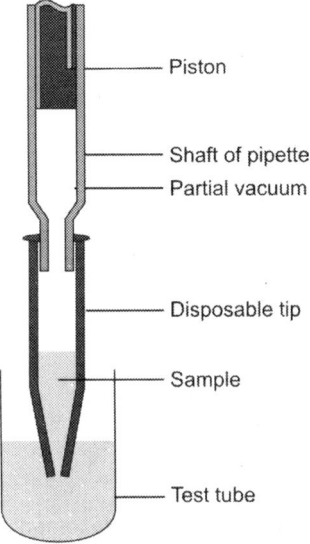

Figure A3.3: Air displacement pipette (ADP)

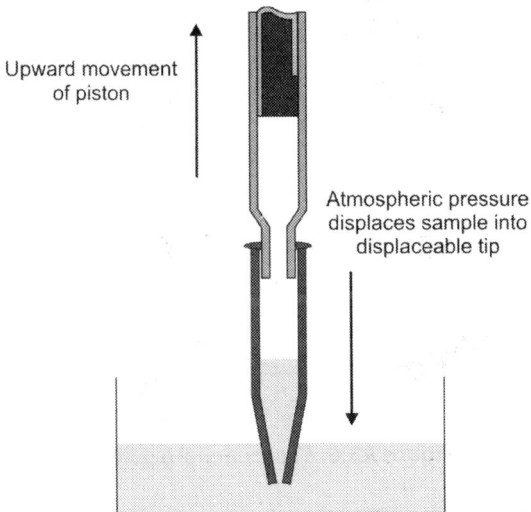

Figure A3.4: Working phenomena of ADP

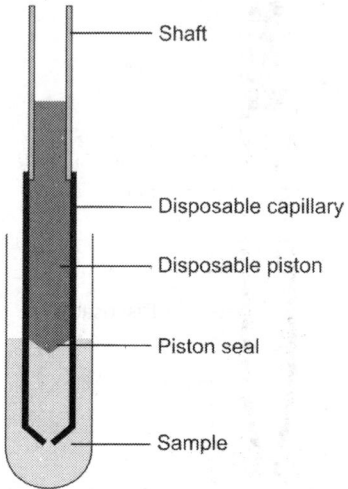

Shaft

Disposable capillary

Disposable piston

Piston seal

Sample

Figure A3.5: Positive displacement pipette

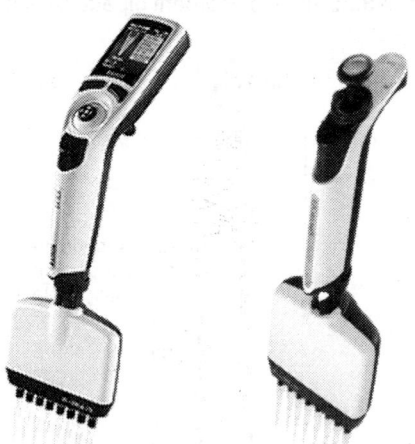

Figure A3.6: Multichannel pipette

11. *Repeater pipette:* These pipettes are used for repeated dispense of equal volume of aliquots after aspiration of a large volume of the liquid. They work based on the principle of positive-displacement. They available both in manual and electronic format.

12. *High throughput pipetting system:* This pipetting system are highly efficient system for delivery of exact amount of liquid to multiple wells at once such as dispensing to 96 wells in ELISA test. They are time efficient and very accurate. Generally they are based on robotic system. But manually operated High throughput pipetting systems are also available.

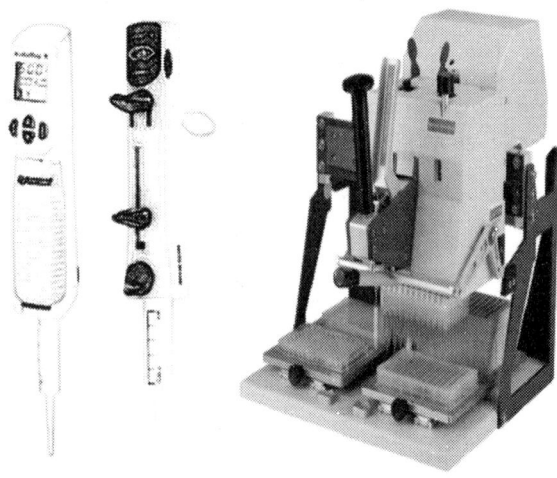

Figure A3.7: High throughput pipetting system

13. *Microfluidic pipette:* It is a recently developed pipette which involves integrates pipetting with microfluidics. This pipetting system is developed by Alar Ainla. Commercially this pipette is known as multifunctional pipette. The pipettes are made from Polydimethylsiloxane (PDMS) is used to manufacture these pipettes.

PIPETTE CONTROLLERS

Different types of pipette controllers are used for aspiration and dispensing of liquid using pipette. These are given below.

1. Manual propipetter bulb is based on squeezing the bulb that attached to the pipette.

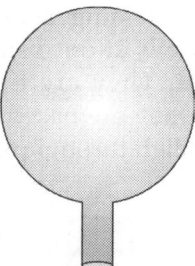

2. Manual propipetter is operated by turning the wheel to aspirate required volume of liquid exactly.

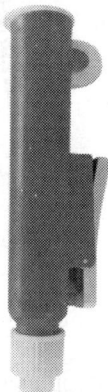

3. Automatic propipetter is used to adjust the volume of the liquid by pressing the button and toggling the switch.

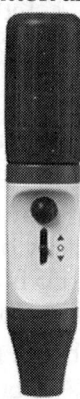

4. Automatic propipetter is used to adjust the volume of the liquid by pulling and pressing the tigger.

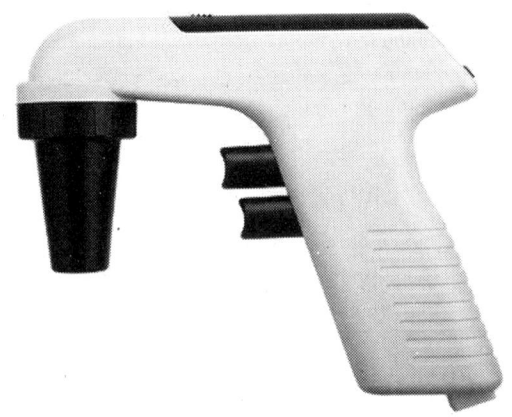

IMPORTANT INSTRUCTIONS FOR HANDLING OF PIPETTE

1. Pipettes should be clean and dry before use,
2. Keep your fingertip dry,
3. It is convenient to use index finger for better control of pipette,
4. Donot hold the pipette between marks because the body temperature may expand the liquid inside the pipette,
5. Wipe off outside of the pipette with tissue paper after dipping in a solution to remove the droplets of liquid adhered on the outside surface of the pipette. Do not touch the tip of pipette with tissue paper,
6. Always keep the pipette vertical to earth surface and mark should be horizontal to eyes during transfer of liquid,
7. Whatever liquid comes out automatically (except blowout pipette) is the actual capacity of the pipette. For volumetric pipette, place the pipette tip in contact with sidewall of the container for full drainage but do not blow out and
8. For better cleaning of pipette, keep pipette in a solution of chromic acid or Triton X-100 before washing.

TOLERANCES ON CAPACITY FOR PIPETTES AS PER INDIAN STANDARDS

1. *For Single Pipettes*

Sl. No.	Nominal capacity (ml)	Tolerance (± ml)	
		Class A	Class B
1	1	0.01	0.02
2	2	0.01	0.02
3	5	0.02	0.03
4	10	0.02	0.04
5	20	0.03	0.05
6	25	0.03	0.06
7	50	0.04	0.08
8	100	0.06	0.12

2. *Graduated Pipettes*

Sl. No.	Nominal capacity (ml)	Subdivision (ml)	Tolerance (± ml)	
			Class A	Class B
1	1	0.01	0.006	0.02
2	2	0.02	0.01	0.06
3	5	0.05	0.03	0.10
4	10	0.10	0.05	0.15
5	25	0.20	0.1	–

Bibliography

1. Schnaare RL, Prince SJ. Remington: *Essentials of Pharmaceutics*. 1st ed. Felton LA, editor. UK: The Pharmaceutical Press; 2013.
2. Ansel HC. *Pharmaceutical Calculations*. 14th ed. Philadelphia: Wolters Kluwer: Lippincott Williams and Wilkins; 2013.
3. Carter SJ, editor. *Tutorial Pharmacy*. 1st ed. India: CBS Publishers and Distributors pvt. Ltd.; 2005.
4. Allen LV, Popovich NG, Ansel HC. Ansel's Pharmaceutical Dosage Forms and Drug Delivery systems. 9th ed. USA: Lippincott Williams and Wilkins; 2015.
5. Sinko PJ, Singh Y, editors. Martin' *Physical Physical Pharmacy and Pharmaceutical Sciences*. 6th ed.: Lippincott Williams and Wilkins; 2011.
6. Rawlins EA, editor. *Bentley's Textbook of Pharmaceutics*. 8th ed.: Elsevier; 2010.
7. Lachman L, Lieberman HA. *The Theory and Practice of Industrial Pharmacy*. 2nd ed.: CBS Publishers and Distributors Pvt. Ltd.; 2011.
8. Sembulingam K, Prema S. *Essentials of Medical Physiology*. 5th ed. New Delhi: Jaypee Brothers Medical Publishers (P) Ltd; 2011.
9. Sahu SN. *Preparation and Distribution of Drugs and Cosmetics*. 1st ed. Ranchi: Kislay Book House; 1990.
10. Indian Pharmacopoiea. 2nd ed. New Delhi: Indian Pharma-copoiea Commission; 1966.
11. Niazi SK. *Handbook of Pharmaceutical Manufacturing Formulations*. 2nd ed. New York: Informa Healthcare USA, Inc.; 2009.
12. *Indian Pharmacopoiea*. 1st ed. New Delhi: Indain Pharma-copoeia Commission; 1955.
13. The Pharmaceutical Society of Great Britain. British Pharmaceutical codex London: The Pharmaceutical Press; 1968.

14. The Pharmaceutical Society of Great Britain. British Pharmaceutical codex London: The Pharmaceutical Press; 1973.
15. British Pharmacopoiea Commission. British Pharmacopoiea. London: Her Majesty's Stationary Office; 1988.
16. The Pharmaceutical Society of Great Britain. British Pharmaceutical Codex. 11th ed. London: The Pharmaceutical Press; 1979.
17. The International Systems of Units (SI), 8th ed.; The BIPM and the Metre Convention: Paris, 2006.
18. Taylor, B. N., Ed. The International System of Units; National Institute of Standards and Technology: Gaithersburg, 2008.
19. Cockcroft, D. W.; Gault, M. *Prediction of Creatinine Clearance from Serum Creatinine. Nephron* 1976, 16, 31–41.
20. Schwartz, G.; Haycock, G.; Edelmann, C.; Spitzer, A. A simple estimate of glomerular filtration rate in children derived from body length and plasma creatinine. *Pediatrics* 1976, 58 (2), 259–263.
21. Jellifee, R. W. Creatinine Clearance: Bedside Estimate. Annals of *Internal Medicine Logo* 1973, 79 (4), 604–605.
22. Sanaka, M.; Takano, K.; Shimakura, K.; Koike, Y.; Mineshita, S. Serum albumin for estimating creatinine clearance in the elderly with muscle atrophy. *Nephron* 1996, 73 (2), 137–144.
23. Salazar, D.; Corcoran, G. Predicting creatinine clearance and renal drug clearance in obese patients from estimated fat-free body mass. *The American Journal of Medicine* 1988, 84 (6), 1053–1060.
24. Greger R. *Units Used in Physiology and Their Definitions.* In: Greger R., Windhorst U. (eds) Comprehensive Human Physiology. Springer, Berlin, 1996.

Index